FRANÇOISE BARBIRA FREEDMAN

yoga for
pregnancy
birth and beyond

LONDON, NEW YORK, MELBOURNE, MUNICH and DELHI

For Lucia, my inspiration for Birthlight

Project Editor Susannah Steel
Art Editor Claire Legemah
Project Art Editor Sara Robin
Managing Editor Gillian Roberts
Managing Art Editor Karen Sawyer
Art Director Carole Ash
Category Publisher Mary-Clare Jerram
DTP Designer Sonia Charbonnier
Production Controller Stuart Masheter
Photographer Russell Sadur

First published in Great Britain in 2004
by Dorling Kindersley Ltd
80 Strand, London WC2R 0RL
Penguin Group (UK)

The reader should not regard the practices described in this
book as substitutes for the advice of a qualified medical
practitioner. Always consult your doctor before starting a
fitness regime if you have any health concerns.

A CIP catalogue record for this book is
available from The British Library

ISBN 1 4053 0056 6

Colour reproduced in Italy by GRB Editrice
Printed and bound in Singapore by
Star Standard Industries (Pte.) Ltd.

Discover more at
www.dk.com

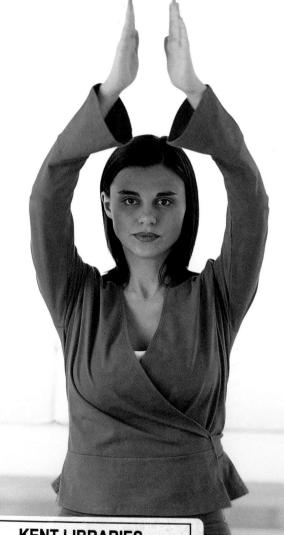

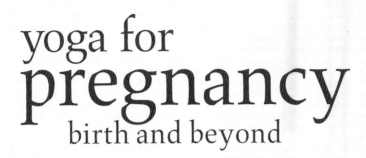

yoga for
pregnancy
birth and beyond

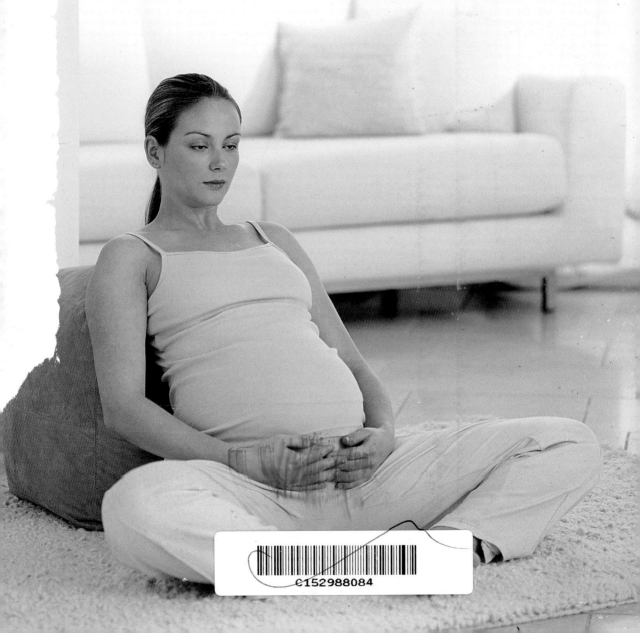

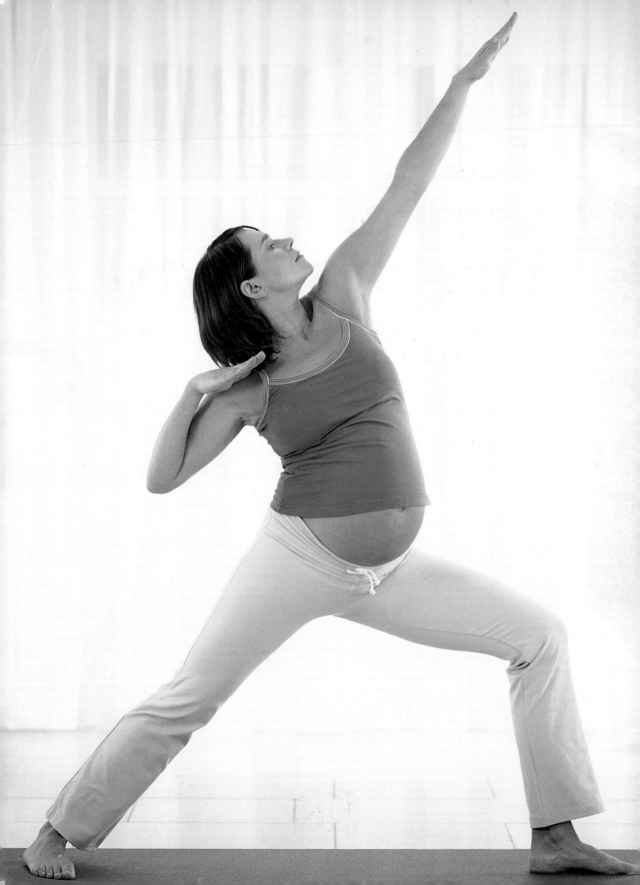

CONTENTS

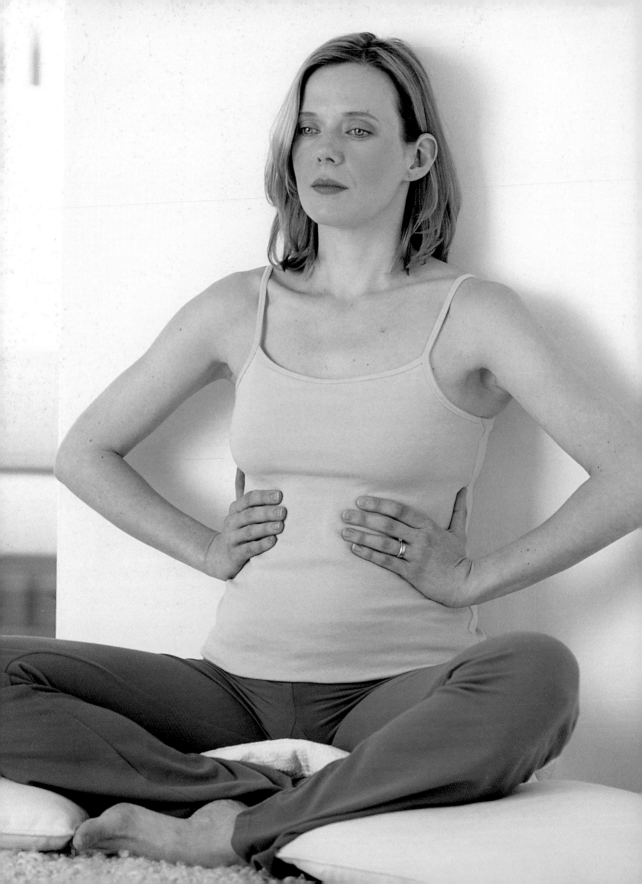

YOGA
FOUNDATIONS

The ancient self-help system of yoga promotes mental and physical well-being and balance, which is vital during times of transition or uncertainty. Your experience of being pregnant and giving birth will involve great physical and emotional changes, and knowing how to use and adapt yoga techniques to breathe, move and relax during this time will help you to lay deep foundations for decades of mothering.

"Grace, beauty, strength, energy and firmness adorn the body through yoga."
Yoga Sutra III, 47

WHY YOGA IN PREGNANCY?

Becoming a mother is a very personal adventure. Although doctors and midwives carefully monitor your health and your baby's growth through pregnancy, yoga brings a calm strength and inner balance that enables you to overcome whatever challenges lie ahead. Whether you are an accomplished yogini, a gym addict, or new to exercise, you will find that yoga is a wonderful and valuable asset in pregnancy.

Adapting classic yoga poses to suit pregnancy can vary between different schools of yoga, but they all stress the importance of relaxation, and precautions for safety. In this book, particular care is given to the first stage of pregnancy when, however fit and experienced you may be, gentle yoga is better than strenuous exercise. As your baby grows, yoga is used to strengthen, tone and relax you, and make more space for your baby.

TONING YOUR MUSCLES

Your pelvic floor muscles, which form a multiplex "hammock" of muscles attached to your lower back and abdominal muscles, require specific training to give your

LOCATING YOUR PELVIC FLOOR

The pelvic floor muscles stretch right across the base of the body, from pubic bone to coccyx, and hold all the abdominal organs in place.

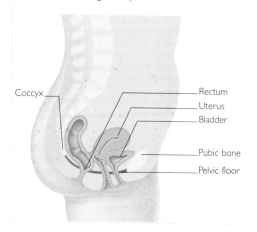

Coccyx

Rectum
Uterus
Bladder

Pubic bone
Pelvic floor

uterus and other organs optimal support in pregnancy. Deep breathing and exercises prepare these muscles to become "birthing muscles" by increasing their elasticity. You will learn to recognize, isolate and activate different muscle groups so that you can use them most effectively during the birth. Your aim is to "birth lightly" – making use of your breath to control these muscles and increase the efficacy of uterine contractions while keeping the rest of your body relaxed. Whatever individual needs you have during the birth, this yoga practice will allow you to release any fear and tension as your baby is born.

THE POWER OF DEEP BREATHING

Toning with your breath is the main focus of the adapted yoga in this book. Your breath is one of yoga's main tools of discovery and connection; with it, you become increasingly self-aware and step lightly through the life-changing experience of motherhood.

Rather than rely on willpower to feel in control during pregnancy and birth, use yoga to help you listen to your body and respond calmly. Relaxation with deep breathing is an effective way to soothe discomforts or disturbing emotions early on before they require further intervention. A greater awareness of your breathing rhythms as you stretch and relax also nurtures you, creating a sense of well-being and contentment that extends through you to your baby, your partner and your family.

The benefits of yoga can continue long after the birth, when deep breathing is used to tone your pelvic floor into peak condition and keep your energies in balance as you adjust to the demands of caring for your newborn.

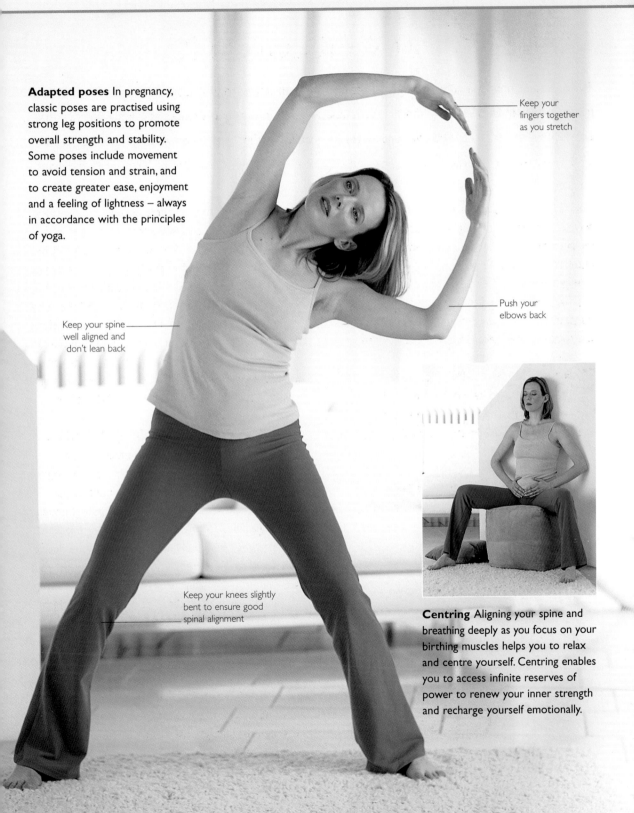

Adapted poses In pregnancy, classic poses are practised using strong leg positions to promote overall strength and stability. Some poses include movement to avoid tension and strain, and to create greater ease, enjoyment and a feeling of lightness – always in accordance with the principles of yoga.

Keep your fingers together as you stretch

Push your elbows back

Keep your spine well aligned and don't lean back

Keep your knees slightly bent to ensure good spinal alignment

Centring Aligning your spine and breathing deeply as you focus on your birthing muscles helps you to relax and centre yourself. Centring enables you to access infinite reserves of power to renew your inner strength and recharge yourself emotionally.

STAGES OF PREGNANCY

The duration of a pregnancy is usually divided into three trimesters, each consisting of three months, and a fourth, postnatal trimester. However, for the purposes of yoga practice, this book is divided by weeks into four stages, which correspond more closely to changes and adjustments experienced by most women.

EARLY PREGNANCY (ONE TO 16 WEEKS)

Less is best in these first weeks as you adapt to hormonal changes and your baby undergoes the most rapid and crucial early formation of the nervous system. Rather than sticking to your usual fitness routine, step back and discover the power of deep breathing as you kneel, sit or lie down. When you feel overcome by fatigue, use yoga to rest deeply and surrender to change with a positive attitude. Developing breath awareness in this relaxed state will enable you to use breathing as a powerful tool to banish anxiety during this intense and delicate period of transformation for both you and your baby.

MID PREGNANCY (16 TO 34 WEEKS)

Once the placenta becomes fully functional, hormone levels balance out and your pregnancy is well established. This is the time to focus on building strength and stamina, aligning your spine at all times and making space for

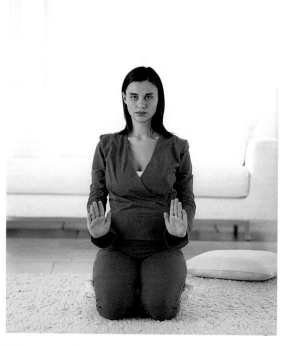

Self-nurture Slow movements, accompanied by the flow of your breath, create a grounding and nurturing effect in early pregnancy, and promote calm strength in stillness.

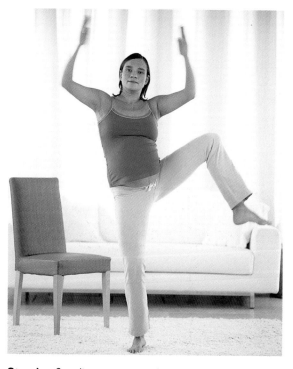

Stamina Standing poses in mid pregnancy provide all-over strengthening for your body. They give a wonderful feeling of vitality while taking pressure off your lower back.

two to "breathe" as your baby grows up towards your rib cage. Most of all, this is the time to enjoy your pregnancy. Yoga will give you energy, strength and agility, expand your breathing capacity and help you to find the right balance between activity and rest. As you sense the first, fluttering movements of your baby, yoga can become a focus for you to develop a receptiveness and connection with this miraculous feat of life inside you.

LATE PREGNANCY (34 TO 40+ WEEKS)

In these last weeks you experience a greater heaviness and a need to focus on the birth. As priorities change, so the aim of yoga now is to keep you comfortable and prepare you physically, mentally and spiritually for labour. Energetic movements alternate with supported stretches and longer periods of deep breathing and relaxation. As you continue to tone your pelvic floor muscles, you

train yourself to be open and without fear. Meanwhile, your baby should respond well to your deep breathing and rotating hip movements as you encourage his or her optimal positioning for birth.

POSTNATAL (BIRTH TO 16 WEEKS)

However you feel after your baby's birth, regaining good posture will be your priority. Your abdominal muscles, which have been very stretched in late pregnancy and may have been cut for the birth, must heal and be strengthened: deep breathing in supported poses is your best ally in toning the muscles of your lower back and abdomen. A safe progression of gentle, adapted poses helps to avoid the strain of too much exercise too soon, which can be counterproductive, while relaxation techniques through the day help you to make up for lost sleep and calmly adjust to life with your new baby.

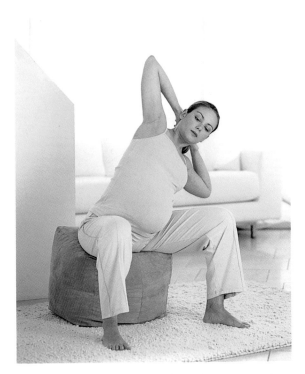

Inner power Seated yoga stretches in late pregnancy keep the base of your body free from tension. This prepares you for bearing down lightly in labour using effective breathing.

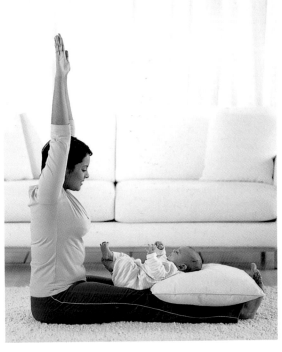

Toning After the joy of welcoming your baby into the world, use the power of your breath to tone the deepest muscles and regain both your figure and a strong back.

FOUNDATIONS OF PRACTICE

The principles of classic yoga – a good alignment of the spine from a solid leg base, and relaxed stretching intensified by deep breathing involving inner muscles – form the basis of every pose in this book. Your strong leg base gradually becomes lower and wider as your baby grows larger, while the gentle yet powerful action of your breathing stretches you in a surprisingly effective and safe way. Most of all, you want to feel relaxed and energized, and enjoy a balance between dynamic and restful poses.

APPLICATION Your body is your best guide: omit exercises that feel uncomfortable or cause pain, and stop if you have had enough. Your heart and lungs are already working at increased levels, so your routine should not be strenuous. Relaxed stretching with breathing expands your breathing capacity without ever exerting force.

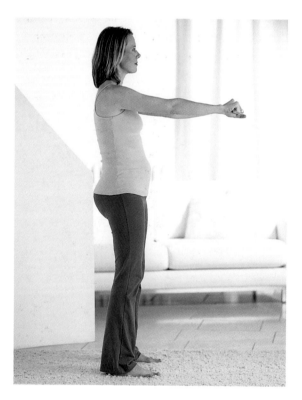

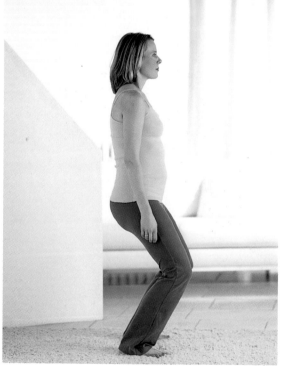

Standing strong In this basic pose your feet are positioned hip-width apart to ensure that your legs are strong and steady. Keep your buttock muscles tensed as you stand up straight. When you exhale, you should feel your abdominal muscles draw in.

Release When you exhale and release, you relax your arms at your sides and let yourself drop by bending your knees. Breathe all the way down your spine, which must remain aligned. This exercise helps you to identify the strong yet relaxed stance of Mountain pose *(p.42)*.

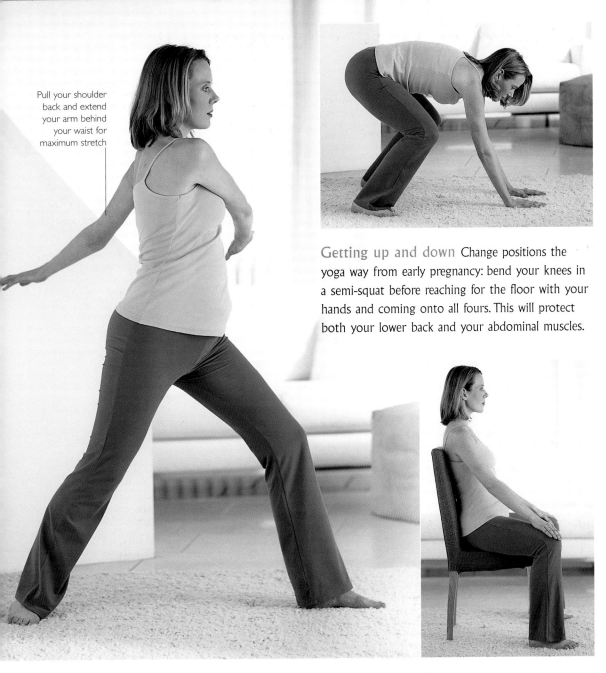

Pull your shoulder back and extend your arm behind your waist for maximum stretch

Getting up and down Change positions the yoga way from early pregnancy: bend your knees in a semi-squat before reaching for the floor with your hands and coming onto all fours. This will protect both your lower back and your abdominal muscles.

Diagonal twists Many classic yoga twists are not advisable during pregnancy due to the pressure they create in the abdomen. Instead, loose diagonal twists relieve tension from the tail bone to the shoulders and neck. Practised rhythmically with the knees slightly bent and the feet wide apart, they create more space for your baby under your rib cage.

Sitting tall Sit upright on a chair with your legs wide apart and your feet firmly on the floor to align your spine and practise deep breathing at all stages of pregnancy.

Relaxed stretch All yoga stretches involve the skeletal muscles, in particular the two deepest layers of muscle. By relaxing the outer layers of muscle, which are usually tensed in action, you can discover how to stretch further. As you stretch, keep all your joints relaxed to feel the extension through your body, and breathe from deep in your pelvis so that your breathing is more effective.

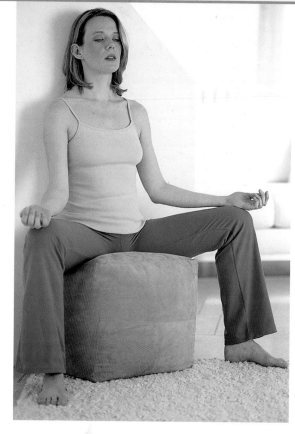

Active relaxation Focused deep breathing in a relaxed, open sitting position helps you to prepare for birth from within and to release tension throughout the pregnancy. Sit with your knees wide apart and your feet firmly planted on the floor. Ensure that your head, shoulders, back and tail bone all remain in contact with the wall as you breathe in and draw up your pelvic floor muscles, then breathe out and release them.

WHY VISUALIZE?

During relaxation or meditation, your focus will probably become more intense. Visualization can help you select a positive, enjoyable focus that induces feelings of calmness and well-being. Images drawn from personal experience are the most powerful. Use visualization to deepen your relaxation and keep anxious thoughts at bay so that you can develop a greater awareness of yourself and your baby.

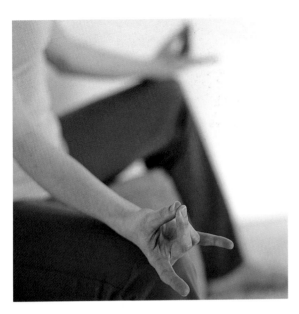

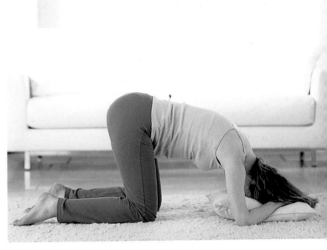

Mudras Subtle positioning of the hands has been a yogic tradition since ancient times. Mudras create specific internal adjustments, which are said to have physical benefits. Many mudras foster inner strength and confidence. A calm, focused approach and a regular practice will increase their positive effects.

Inner stretch Some yoga poses strengthen muscle groups that we are not usually aware of. Muscles used in childbirth gain from toning and inner stretch. This is achieved by gradually connecting deep breathing with muscular action. Being on all fours reduces the pull of gravity on these muscles as you tone them.

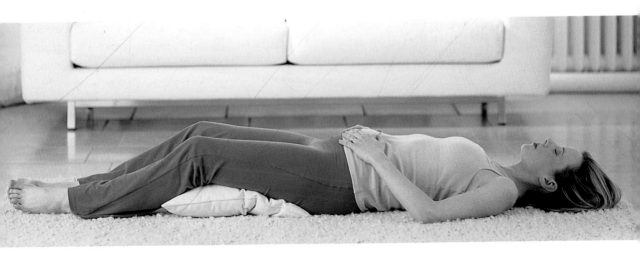

Deep relaxation Always leave enough time to end every yoga practice, however short, with deep relaxation. The classic Corpse pose, to which you can add various supports for necessary comfort before and after birth, balances activity with rest in minimal time. Relaxation opens a space in which you can nurture your emotional bond with your baby long before birth, and grow in your unconditional love.

HOW TO USE THIS BOOK

Yoga is rooted in experience, so your yoga practice before, during and after the birth should – above all – suit your individual needs and lifestyle. Select yoga exercises that match your own level of fitness, your timetable, and even your mood, to create a unique yoga routine. After you have read these guidelines, you are ready to begin your practice.

Classic yoga poses are carefully adapted in this book to assist the transition to motherhood. They include a steady progression of skills, in particular the use of breathing and relaxed stretching. Each spread illustrates a complete sequence as a ready-made practice. However, there are no set routines in this book. You can pick out individual poses from one spread and combine them with different poses from other spreads as you wish, or to suit your available time or energy levels.

If you begin this book in mid or late pregnancy, use the whole book rather than just your relevant section, as earlier exercises may give you the foundations you need now. If you are a keen practitioner of yoga, don't under-estimate some of the adapted poses; their simplicity will help you to deepen your breathing and your practice as your body and mind change through the months.

A regular practice every day, no matter how short, is best to ensure that yoga not only tones and refreshes you, but also opens up a space in your day for you to quietly welcome your baby and let yourself be. In fact, many of the exercises can be integrated into your daily routine, wherever you are. Use them to develop a better posture as you stand, walk, sit at a desk or clean the house. Alternatively, select an exercise for an "instant" practice if you have only a few minutes to spare.

Creating a yoga corner at home is conducive to a regular practice. Keep your props there (including a yoga belt, yoga blocks and cushions), and check that you have a solid chair with an upright back to hand. Ensure that you practise yoga on a firm, non-slip, comfortable surface – either a carpet, rug or yoga mat – and always

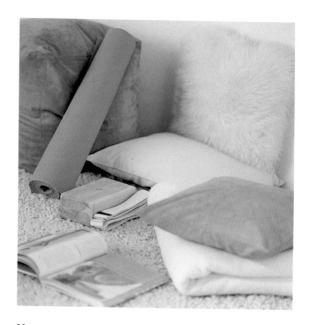

Yoga space Create a yoga corner for yourself, even if it is just somewhere to unroll a yoga mat. You will need props such as a pouffe or bean bag, a flat cushion to place under your head, two fuller cushions and a shawl for relaxation.

practise a pose on both sides of your body. If you are new to yoga, the guidelines listed here will help you to make up your own balanced, harmonious yoga practice.

STARTING POSE
Take a few breaths in a starting pose to set your intent to engage in a sequence of moves: Mountain pose *(p.42)* for standing yoga poses and yoga dance; Sitting square *(p.32)* for sitting poses; Cat pose *(p.67)* for kneeling stretches; and Aligned supine pose *(p.20)* for poses on your back.

GROUNDING

Depending on your starting pose and which stage of pregnancy you are at, select one or more exercises that either stretch you dynamically (for example, Sun salutations – either complete or in part – Circular stretches, Standing twists, Kneeling rolls, Sitting stretches), or stretch you in a relaxed way (Spinal rolls, Supported sitting stretches, Active relaxation). As well as warming you up, these stretches help you to breathe with each movement and engage your mind.

EXPANSION

Include one or more poses that correspond to your stage of pregnancy. You may wish to explore adapted versions of classic poses (such as the Thunderbolt *(pp.24–25)*, Tree pose *(pp.60–61)*, Archer to Warrior pose *(pp.54–57)*, or Moon pose *(p.51, p.53)*), or practise a special application to relieve a particular condition. Alternatively, you can make breathing your main practice with a focus on diaphragmatic breathing (such as Breath awareness).

INTEGRATION

As you focus on what your body and breath are doing, your mind becomes still and centred. This integrated focus absorbs not only the normal flurry of thoughts, but also intense emotions; yoga draws your energies into balance and connects you with a deeper steadiness. Use Spinal alignments, Hip openers, Shoulder stretches, toning the pelvic muscles, Sitting stretches or Active relaxation. Hand movements, or Mudras, and breathing techniques are also conducive to an integration of breathing, movement and awareness.

RELAXATION

Allow at least three minutes relaxation time to complete your practice. Relaxation is essential as it enables you to gain the physiological benefits brought about by deep breathing and stretching. Try sitting poses, Supported inversions, Forward bends, Corpse pose and Walking relaxation. These will also help during labour and beyond, renewing your energy levels and calming your baby.

Modifying your practice If the circumstances are not right for you to do yoga – for example, after a meal or late at night – a few minutes of deep breathing followed by relaxation are most beneficial.

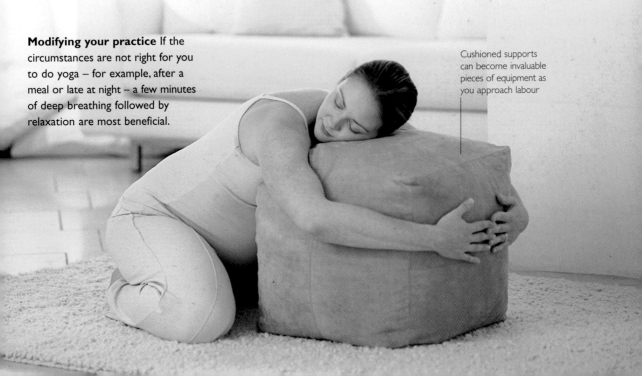

Cushioned supports can become invaluable pieces of equipment as you approach labour

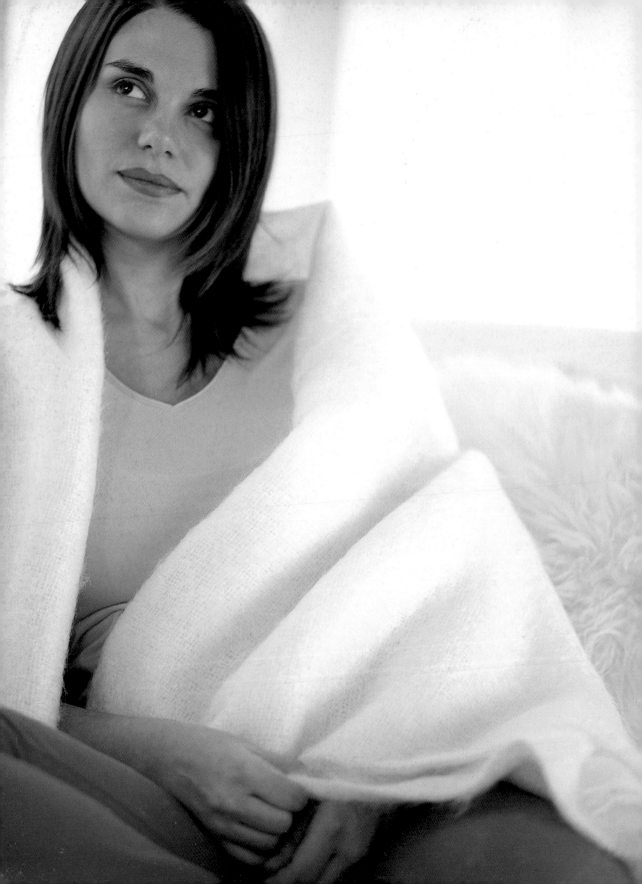

EARLY PREGNANCY

ONE TO 16 WEEKS

Making space in your life for a new baby is now a priority for you,
not only emotionally but physically. You will need to slow down and
discover the power of micro-movement and in-depth relaxed stretches
that avoid any strain in your pelvic area. You also need to learn to
breathe more deeply, relax more effectively and develop an awareness
of your pelvic muscles. In this way you can prepare your spine
and your whole body for the changes of pregnancy.

"It is the growing presence of an embryo
that teaches us our paths are truly joined."
Climbing Sun

BASIC PELVIC ALIGNMENT

Pelvic awareness enables you to adjust and improve your spinal alignment as your body changes through pregnancy. This relaxed sequence develops deep abdominal breathing and tones the whole pelvic area at a very important time in the formation of your baby's main organs. Performing these stretches on your back will draw your attention to the tilt of your pelvis in relation to your spine. Each movement is synchronized to an inhalation or exhalation.

> **BENEFITS** No one is perfectly aligned, and in pregnancy asymmetry may cause lower back pain. Try these curative pelvic stretches if:
> • Your pelvis tilts forwards.
> • You have previously carried a baby or toddler on one hip.
> • You consistently rest your weight on one leg.

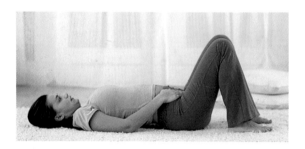

1 Lie on your back with your knees bent and slightly apart, and your feet flat and aligned with your knees. Ensure that your whole spine is in contact with the floor so that your neck is comfortable. Place your hands loosely on your lower abdomen.

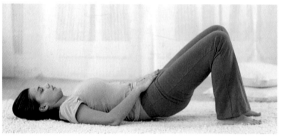

2 Breathe evenly, in and out. As you exhale, press the middle of your back onto the floor. Repeat several times. Your tail bone may lift slightly as your abdominal breathing deepens, so try to make more contact with the floor on each exhalation.

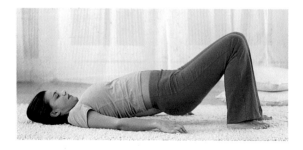

3 Press the palms of your hands onto the floor, lift your hips slightly and move your pelvis from side to side with micro-movements. If this is easy and pain-free, move in a few small clockwise, then anti-clockwise, circles. Then rest and breathe deeply.

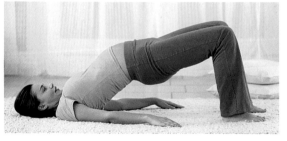

4 If you feel ready for more, breathe in and push your hips up high. As you exhale slowly, lower your body down so that you elongate your back as much as possible. Repeat twice with a short rest in between each stretch.

5 Now take an in-breath and lift your hips off the floor again. As you exhale this time, lift your right hip and let your left hip drop. Inhale and stretch on the other side, lifting the left hip and dropping the right hip. Repeat three times, registering any difference between the stretches on either side of your body. Then rest and breathe deeply with your back aligned on the floor.

Lift your right hip up and drop your left hip down at the same time

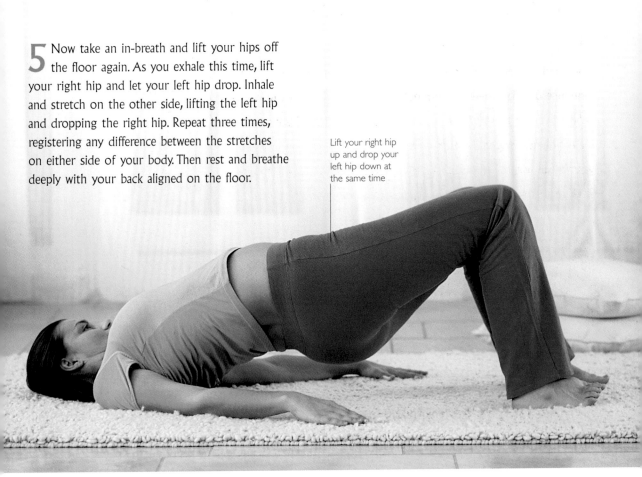

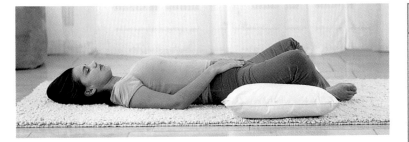

6 End this sequence with a relaxation. Place a cushion under your thighs to ensure that your lower back is in contact with the floor. Let your knees flop outwards. If this feels comfortable, bring the soles of your feet together in Butterfly pose. After a few deep breaths, let go of any tension to enhance the blood circulation to your pelvic area.

RELAX IN THE POSE

- Do not open your knees during your relaxation unless they are fully supported by your cushion.
- Place a flat cushion under your neck and head if you want to feel more comfortable.
- Use another cushion if needed to support your feet in Butterfly pose.
- Take time to nurture the space in which your baby is growing. Relaxing is a physical expression of your care for your baby growing inside you.

SPINAL ROLLS

This floor sequence combines stretching and relaxation using rolling movements. These flowing poses, which you can practise at your own fast or slow pace, adapt yoga twists and bends in a safe way for pregnancy, with a focus on relaxed yet deep toning of the abdominal and lower back muscles. You can practise these rolls throughout pregnancy and beyond: they will help you to sleep better in late pregnancy and to have fun with your baby after the birth.

BENEFITS AND CAUTIONS

These rolls relieve tension in the neck and head, and are preventative and curative poses for sciatic pain.

If you have had abdominal surgery or a Caesarean section less than two years ago, rest your feet on the floor for the Twisting rolls.

TWISTING ROLL

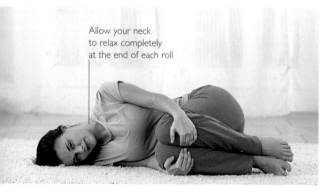

Allow your neck to relax completely at the end of each roll

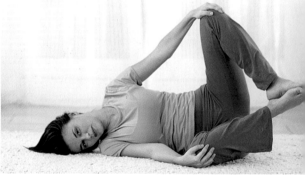

1 Lie on your back with your knees bent and your hands gently holding your knees. As you exhale, flop your knees over to the right and roll softly onto your right side. Inhale, roll onto your back again and repeat on the left side. Repeat four times, then rest.

2 Lie on your back with your hands on your bent knees. Open your knees wide and inhale. Try to join the soles of your feet in Butterfly pose. Exhale and roll onto your right side, keeping your neck relaxed. Inhale and roll onto your back. Repeat on the left side.

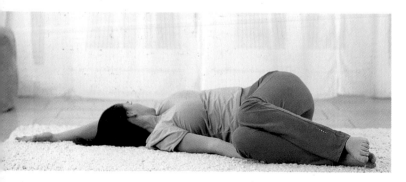

3 Add a yoga twist to step 1 after you have dropped your knees and rolled to the right: extend your left arm along the floor, as close to your head as possible, in a relaxed stretch. Breathe deeply in this diagonal stretch before changing sides. Repeat twice.

LONG STRETCH ROLL

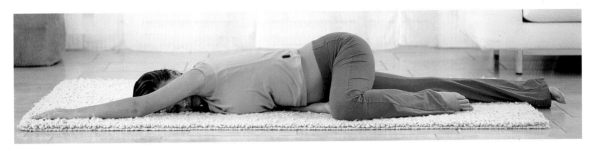

1 Lie on your right side with your legs bent and your hands on your knees (as in step 1 of Twisting roll) and inhale. As you exhale, keep your left leg and right arm in position while you extend your left arm out along the floor and straighten your right leg. Practise this sequence very slowly on each side. Allow your abdominal breathing to deepen in this relaxed diagonal stretch before moving on to step 2.

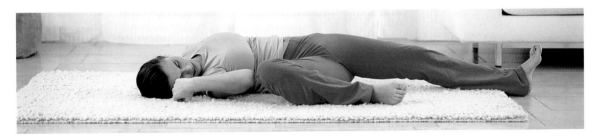

2 Lying on your right side, inhale and roll onto your back. Exhale as you relax your left arm and slowly straighten your left leg. Inhale and draw your right knee up to your right elbow. Exhale and roll your left shoulder out so that your upper back makes contact with the floor. Repeat on the left side. When you feel confident, alternate on each side in a flowing motion in time with your breathing.

Keep your arm and shoulder relaxed so that the roll is distributed evenly along the whole spine

Rolls such as this help to avert tension in the neck and shoulders

3 Lie on your back with your legs straight and arms relaxed. Inhale, bend your right leg and roll it over your left leg. As you roll onto your left side, exhale and extend your right arm by your head. To reverse the movement, bend your left leg, straighten your right leg and roll to the right. Thus you bend, stretch, twist and roll in a smooth, harmonious motion to the rhythm of your breathing.

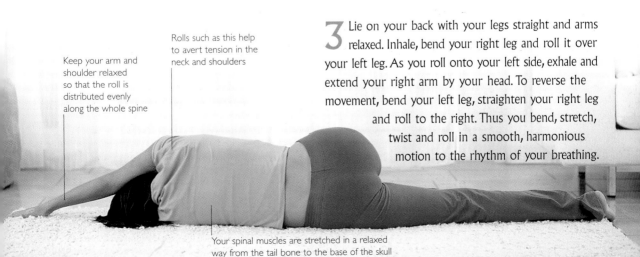

Your spinal muscles are stretched in a relaxed way from the tail bone to the base of the skull

THE THUNDERBOLT
Vajrasana

The two cyclic movements in this classic yoga pose will give you the calm strength and centring you need to face all the intense emotions and changes to your body throughout pregnancy. Discover the power of your breathing as you stretch out, then draw inwards. With practice, you will discover your own rhythms and the pace that best suits you in this pose to make you feel simultaneously energized and relaxed. You should also experience deep muscular toning.

BENEFITS AND CAUTIONS
The Thunderbolt aligns the spine, alleviates back pain and tones the muscles supporting the breasts.

If you have high blood pressure, stop after step 3. If you feel faint or dizzy in Child's pose, rest your head on a chair or sit up slowly.

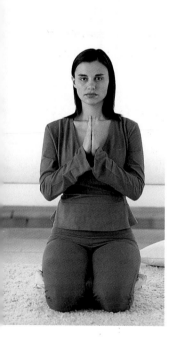
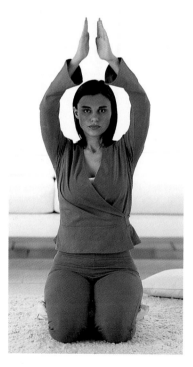
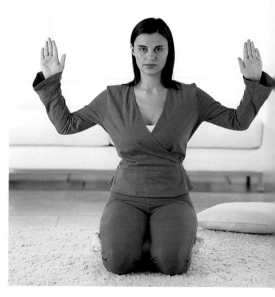

1 Place a cushion between your feet and buttocks and kneel with your back straight. Inhale and join your hands at chest height.

2 Continue to inhale as you lift your hands above your head in Prayer pose. Avoid tensing your shoulders. As you exhale, draw your hands apart without moving your shoulders or elbows.

3 Continue to exhale as you slowly bring your bent arms out in a wide circle until the palms of your hands are facing forwards. Push your elbows out and back. Inhale and exhale again slowly in this position. Repeat in another slow cycle.

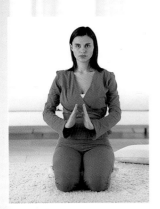

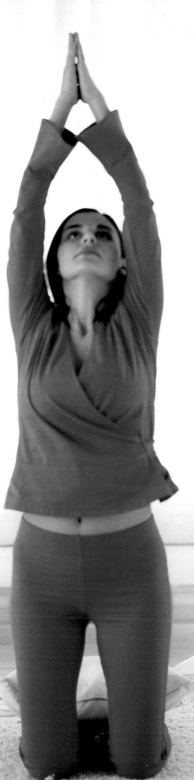

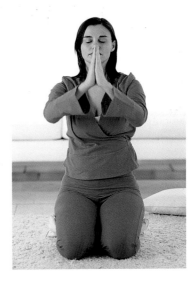

4 This second movement is particularly beneficial for women whose right abdominal muscles have "split" in a previous pregnancy. Align your spine and check that your lower back is neither arched nor collapsed. Join your hands in Prayer pose and keep your elbows down. Inhale, lift up into an upright kneeling position and stretch your arms above your head. Look up at your hands. As your abdominal breathing develops, you will feel this stretch more deeply in your pelvis.

5 Kneel down slowly, keeping your back strong as you exhale and lower your hands. Repeat steps 4 and 5 two or three times.

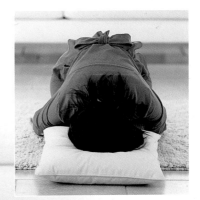

6 Deep rest, an essential component of the two cycles, is best done in Child's pose. As you kneel, open your knees wider to make room for your baby and bend forwards, resting your head on a cushion. Relax your arms on the floor with your palms face up and breathe deeply and slowly.

EASY TRIANGLE
Trikonasana

This classic pose suits both pregnant women who are new to yoga and experienced practitioners who want to get the greatest benefit from the Triangle during their pregnancy. In order to avoid any strain in the held Triangle pose, this sequence begins with relaxed stretches to move your body and loosen your muscles. Then the dynamic stillness of the held pose becomes effortless.

BENEFITS Practise this pose in early pregnancy to help you expand your breathing capacity. Triangle may also help to prevent or relieve heartburn. Whenever you feel tension in the held pose, enjoy the easier rhythmical variations instead.

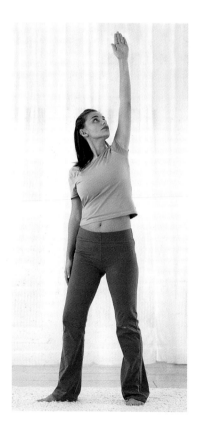

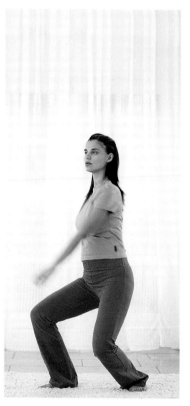

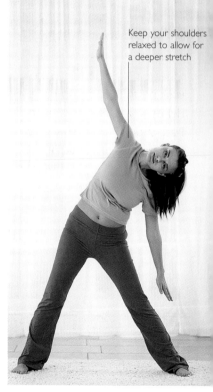

Keep your shoulders relaxed to allow for a deeper stretch

1 Stand with feet hip-width apart and with your right foot turned out. Inhale, raise your left arm and look up at your hand. Exhale and stretch up through your hand.

2 Inhale and circle your left arm. Exhale and bend your knees as your arm drops down, then inhale up to complete the circle. Repeat steps 1 and 2 on the right side.

3 Move your feet further apart and extend your arms out horizontally. Inhale, bend over to the left and exhale. Inhale up and repeat on the other side.

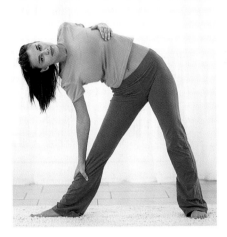

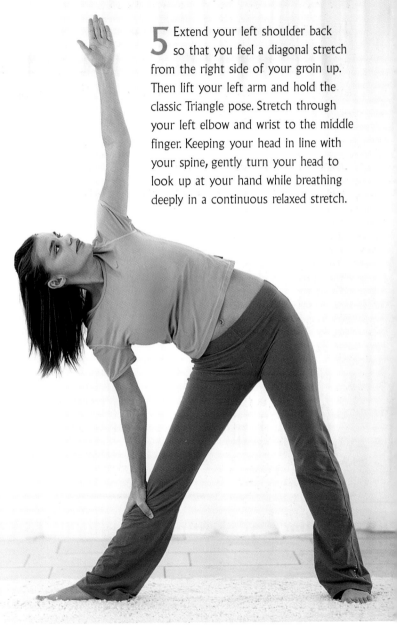

5 Extend your left shoulder back so that you feel a diagonal stretch from the right side of your groin up. Then lift your left arm and hold the classic Triangle pose. Stretch through your left elbow and wrist to the middle finger. Keeping your head in line with your spine, gently turn your head to look up at your hand while breathing deeply in a continuous relaxed stretch.

4 The classic Triangle pose is presented in two progressive steps. Stand with your legs wide apart and with your right foot pointing out. Let your right arm rest anywhere along your right leg that feels most comfortable. Place your left hand on the side of your rib cage in an opening stretch as you breathe deeply in and out.

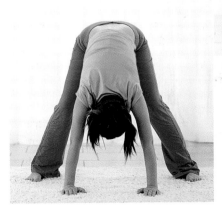

6 Relax in this loose Forward bend. Keep your knees bent and rest your hands on the floor for stability and to gain a deeper stretch in your lower spine. Keep your head relaxed as you take several deep abdominal breaths before either going down onto all fours or standing up slowly.

ADAPTED SHOULDER STANDS
Sarvangasana

The "queen" of classic yoga postures is adapted here so that pregnant women who are new to yoga can receive its benefits without strain. Even if you are an experienced practitioner, it is best to use these easy variations to rest and to deepen your abdominal breathing in early pregnancy. Each variation develops your awareness of the connections between your lower back muscles and abdominal muscles. Use a support to allow for a wide range of adapted poses to suit your individual needs during pregnancy.

BENEFITS Inverted poses such as these stimulate blood circulation in the pelvic area and the legs. Use these supported adaptations:
• To help you rest in the evenings.
• If you work standing up.
• If you have varicose veins or wish to prevent them occurring. Deep breathing in restful poses also helps to calm the emotions.

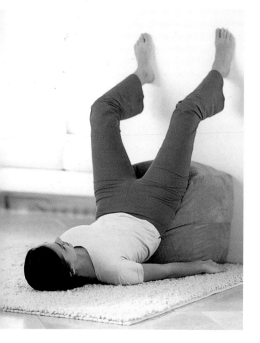

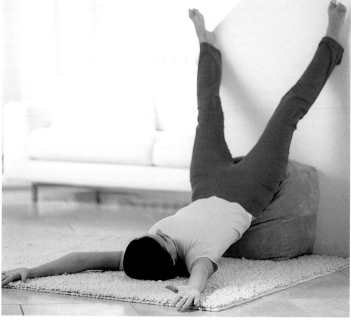

1 Position a bean bag or pouffe against a wall to support your hips, and rest your upper back and head on the floor. Place both feet against the wall, keep your knees bent and rest your arms on the floor. Breathe deeply and relax.

2 This stretch complements step 1 by allowing you to open your chest and abdomen fully. Press your lower back onto your support and stretch into your heels. Extend your arms out along the floor behind your head and stretch into your fingertips. Then practise inhaling lightly, gradually lengthening the time you take to breathe out. Continue for six breaths or more.

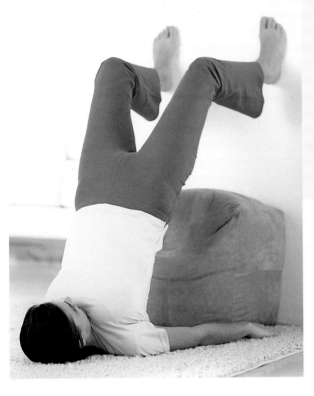

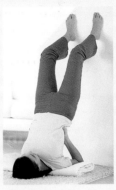

ADVANCED MOVE

If you are familiar with the classic pose, place a folded blanket under your shoulders, lie down and lift your legs on an out-breath. Rest your feet against the wall and support your back with your hands.

3 If you feel confident, push yourself up into an easy Bridge shoulder stand by pressing your feet against the wall and raising your hips right up as you inhale. If you feel comfortable, hold the lift for a few breaths, but ensure that you don't strain your neck or eyes at any time. Lower down onto the pouffe as you slowly exhale.

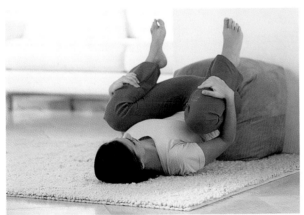

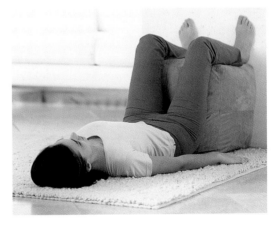

4 Bend your legs and draw your knees up on either side of your chest. Place your hands gently on your shins. As you inhale, draw in the muscles of your lower abdomen and, if you can, your pelvic floor muscles. Relax and exhale. Then slide your hips down onto the floor and relax your arms and legs.

5 Rest and breathe deeply. This is an ideal position in which to feel grounded yet light, centred yet free, whenever you need to refresh your outlook. Keep your legs raised and relaxed. Let go of any worries and take a few moments to silently welcome your baby into your life.

SHOULDER STRETCHES

This dynamic standing sequence of stretches, which open out your chest and loosen your shoulders, is relatively easy to do and can generate a great sense of fun. All these movements are achieved by standing with your knees slightly bent to avoid any arching of the back as you stretch. You can also try these poses while sitting on a stool or kneeling, as in the Thunderbolt pose *(pp.24–25)*. Enjoy practising them whenever you have a free moment in the day.

> **BENEFITS** Try this sequence when you feel tired, as its positive effects may help to lift your mood and energize you. Shoulder stretches also help to:
> • Prevent and relieve heartburn.
> • Maintain a strong posture.
> • Open up your heart area.
> • Ease tension in the shoulders.

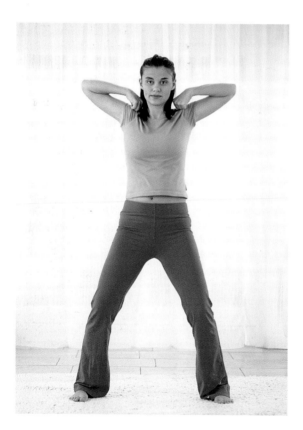

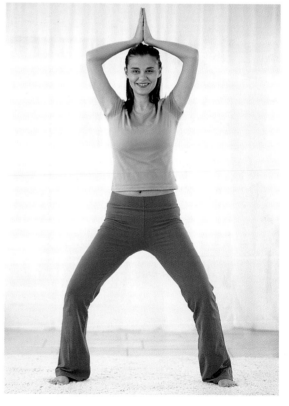

1 Position your feet wide apart and place the knuckles of your hands at the base of your neck. Lift your elbows, inhale and bring your elbows together in front of your chest. Exhale and push them back as far as possible. Repeat this movement several times.

2 Bring your hands together in Prayer pose and position them on top of your head. Push your elbows right back. If this is easy for you, alternately lift each elbow in a rhythm that suits you. Make this movement fun, light-hearted and full of zest.

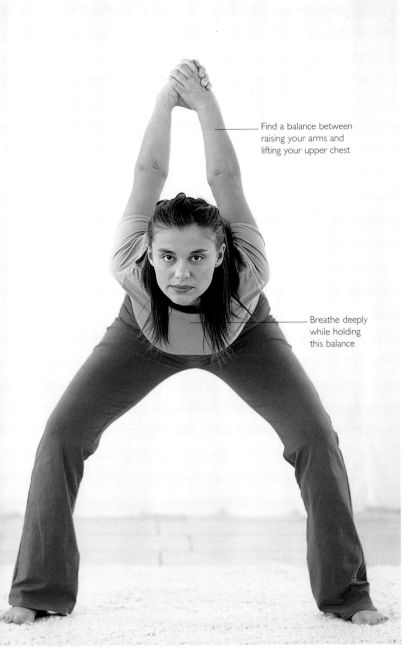

Find a balance between
raising your arms and
lifting your upper chest

Breathe deeply
while holding
this balance

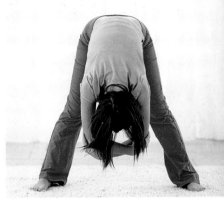

4 Keep your knees bent or, if
you can, straighten your legs.
Relax your arms down, cup your
elbows with your hands and stretch
your shoulders down. Breathe
deeply. If you feel dizzy, stand up.

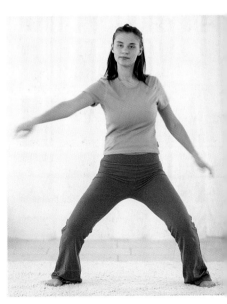

3 Lean forwards from the hips and clasp one wrist behind your back
with your other hand. Keeping your back straight, extend your
arms away from your body. Bend a little lower and turn your knees
out slightly to create more space as you lift your arms and upper
chest and look up. Repeat, clasping the other wrist.

5 Return to a standing position,
keeping your knees bent as
you loosely swing your arms from
side to side and gently wrap them
around your body.

SITTING STRETCHES

These easy sitting stretches help you to gain awareness of the muscle groups that enable you to walk and sit straight as the weight of your growing baby increases each month. This combination of relaxed stretches and twists involving the whole length of your spine is ideal if you sit down to work, or if you need a quick break in a busy day to stretch. The fine toning achieved may surprise even advanced practitioners.

1 Choose a firm seat or stool that enables your knees to be level with, or lower than, your hips. Sit with your legs apart and extend your right arm up slowly as you inhale, keeping your torso and neck relaxed. Stretch into your fingers as you exhale and relax at the end of your out-breath. Repeat with your left arm.

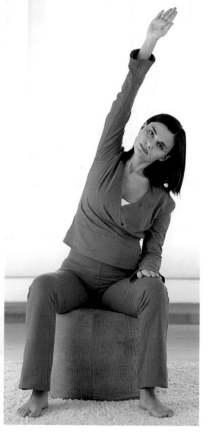

2 Inhale and extend your right arm up. Keeping your hips still, gently move your raised arm over to the left and exhale. Repeat with the left arm.

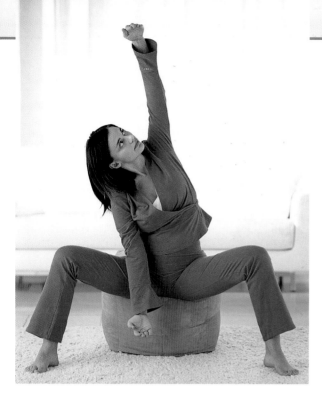

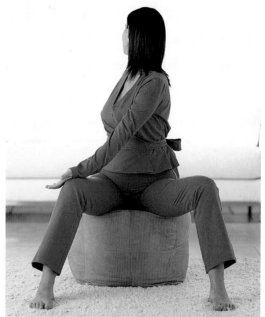

3 Extend the stretch further down the spine: with your knees wide apart and your arms outstretched, gently roll an imaginary globe in your hands. Rotate your torso slowly as your hands roll clockwise, then anticlockwise. Use your imagination to "feel" this large globe.

4 Twist your upper body to the right. Place the back of your left hand on the outside of your right knee and the back of your right hand against your left buttock. Use both hands to extend this twisting movement as you exhale.

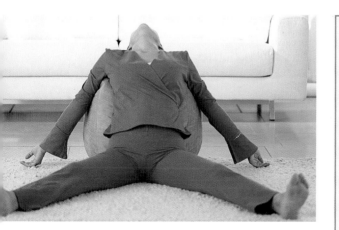

5 Relax by sitting on the floor against your support with your legs wide apart. Lean right back and open your chest fully. Relax your arms and, if it feels comfortable, recline your head on the support.

VISUALIZATION

Cultivate the yogic skill of stretching just one area of your body at a time while the rest of your body remains relaxed. Concentrate on performing each easy sitting position slowly and softly:

• Release your lower back down first and, as you stretch and breathe, be aware of your spine lengthening from the base up.

• Keep your head and facial muscles relaxed throughout this sequence.

• Become aware of stretching the deepest layer of your skeletal muscles effortlessly by using your deep breathing effectively.

• The long muscles along your spine are key to your strength and comfort through pregnancy. Be aware that long before birth, your baby benefits from the support of your strong and supple back.

BREATH & AWARENESS

The action of yoga on our physiology is primarily through breathing and awareness. Without them, poses and movements remain just exercises. Whatever your experience of being pregnant, your awareness of your natural breathing rhythm can help to link your emotions and thoughts to physical sensations. In a state of calm awareness, breathing becomes a powerful tool of transformation.

BREATHING

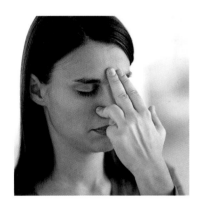

Alternate nostril breathing
Close your eyes and place the index and middle fingers of one hand between your eyebrows. Close one nostril with your thumb and inhale through the open nostril. Close this nostril with your third finger, release your thumb and exhale through the freed nostril. Repeat several times.

BENEFITS These simple practices are effective techniques to link body and spirit through a combination of breathing and expressive gestures. In pregnancy they are particularly useful for:
• Centring yourself and accessing your inner strength.
• Calming yourself instantly using deep breathing.
• Developing your awareness of good alignment. Breathing, mudras and meditation are most effective if your spine is well aligned.
• Nurturing yourself and your baby.
• Increasing your awareness of involuntary tensions and your ability to relax your pelvic floor muscles.
• Helping you discover the power of intent expressed in your gestures.
• Introducing you to the refreshing power of meditation.

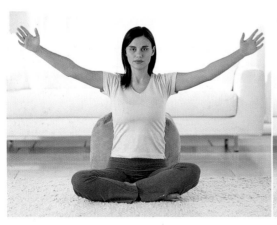
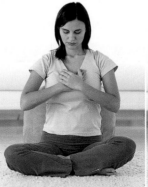
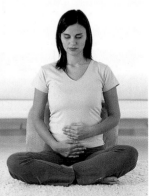

Prana In this slow movement you expand your in-breath to take in prana (universal energy) and direct it to yourself and your baby. Sit on the floor with your back supported and your legs crossed or straight.

Inhale, spread your arms in a wide embrace with your palms open, exhale and cross your hands over your chest. Inhale and rest your hands on your abdomen. Exhale and repeat, deepening your breathing each time.

MUDRAS

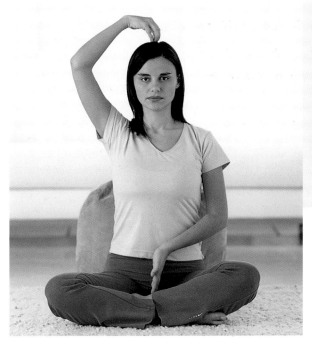

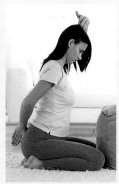

ALTERNATIVE
If a kneeling position feels more comfortable, place your lower hand over your tail bone instead. Elongate your lower spine with a gentle back tilt of your pelvis for four slow exhalations.

Vertical axis Mudras are hand positions that express awareness and intent. Sit on the floor against a support to align your spine. Place the fingers of one hand on your crown and the side of your other hand at your pubic bone. Breathe deeply for four breaths along this vertical axis.

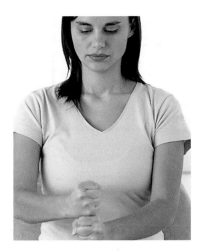

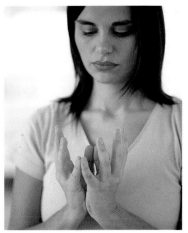

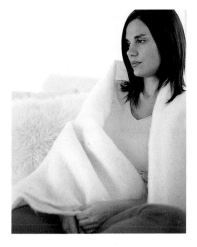

Energy-charging mudra Make fists, one on top of the other with your thumbs out, at elbow height. Breathe deeply without clenching your fists to gather new reserves of calm strength.

Lotus mudra Make the shape of a lotus bud: join the outer edges of each hand and the pads of your little fingers and thumbs. Spread your remaining fingers. Take four deep breaths, then relax.

Meditation Sit quietly to meditate and integrate the effects of the mudras and your breathing practice. A prayer shawl may feel soothing and protective, as well as keep you warm.

RELAX, OPEN, NURTURE

Relaxation is an essential component of your yoga routine, as it allows stretches to take their full effect in your body. The different supported postures shown here will help you to open and nurture yourself in preparation for becoming a mother. Whenever you feel overwhelmed or exhausted by your pregnancy, access the deep relaxation that exists within you and enjoy the presence of your growing baby in a tranquil space.

EYES QUIET

MAHA SACRAL MUDRA

CORPSE POSE

For this relaxation pose, place two cushions under both of your knees to ensure that your whole spine is perfectly aligned. Let your knees softly flop outwards. Place your hands over your lower abdomen and create a triangle by joining your thumbs and index fingers. Close your eyes and be aware of your femininity and of becoming a mother.

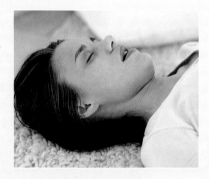

Keep your head straight and your neck relaxed so that you can look straight above you. Close your eyes and quieten their activity as you drop your lower jaw and relax your face. Breathe evenly and effortlessly.

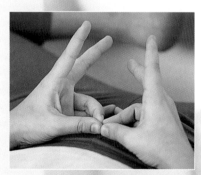

Press the pads of your little fingers together and place the pads of your ring fingers on those of your thumbs. Hold for ten breaths. This large pelvis mudra is known for its relaxing and energy-balancing effect.

Press your lumbar spine onto the floor with a few deep abdominal breaths so that you feel more relaxed

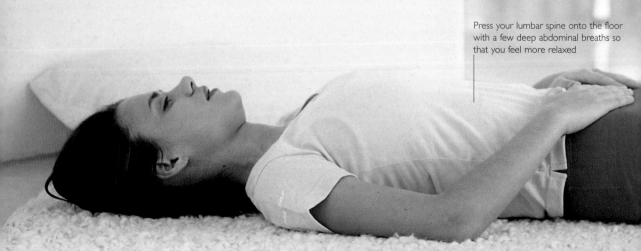

SUPINE BUTTERFLY POSE

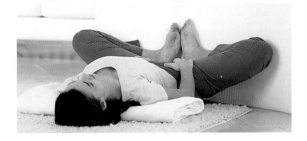

This classic resting Butterfly pose is known for its positive effects on the female reproductive organs. Here it is performed against a wall to help you open your pelvis more easily. Use a folded blanket to give added support to your rib cage and use cushions, if needed, under your knees. Lie on the floor facing the wall. Join the soles of your feet and drop your knees out to the sides, as wide as feels comfortable.

WORK IN THE POSE

• Make sure that you will not be disturbed, then choose your pose and position yourself carefully so that you feel comfortable.
• Don't be discouraged if you can't instantly quieten your mind; practice makes perfect.
• Hold each pose for an average of five to ten minutes, longer if possible. Change position at any time if you feel discomfort.
• Allow a few minutes to relax before performing mudras.
• To return to normal activity, take a few deep breaths, let your eyes open gently and roll onto one side before getting up slowly.

RELAXATION WITH SUPPORTED TORSO

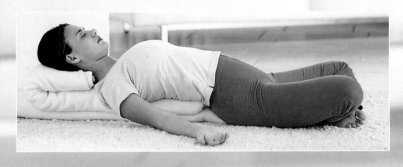

Fold two blankets lengthwise so that they support your upper and lower spine. Fold back one end of the upper blanket so that it can support your head. Lie evenly on the blankets and cross or extend your legs. Relax your arms at your sides with your palms opened out.

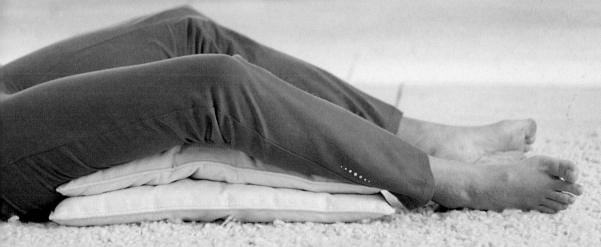

SPECIAL APPLICATIONS

Many women find early pregnancy most challenging. Discomforts associated with hormonal changes, such as exhaustion and nausea, can be alleviated with yoga until they subside later on. However, anxiety, pelvic pain and backache may be longer-lasting, and so require preventative yoga.

Your breath is your main tool in these simple yet effective exercises, which act simultaneously on your endocrine glands and nervous system. The effect of each exercise is cumulative, so that frequent practice through the day brings the best results for each of these conditions.

TIREDNESS

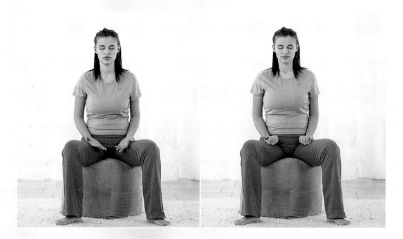

Sit up straight with your knees apart. Place your hands, palms up, against your lower abdomen so that your fingers point towards each other. Breathe in deeply and feel your abdomen expand. Gather energy and slowly breathe in and out for six breaths. Then curl up your fingers, turn your wrists out and breathe intensely in your upper chest for six more breaths.

HEARTBURN

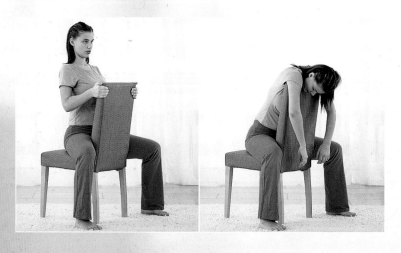

Lifting your sternum and opening out your shoulder blades helps to alleviate heartburn. Sit astride a chair facing backwards and hold onto the chair back with both hands. Pull your shoulders right back and breathe steadily for six breaths. Then flop your arms over the back of the chair, broadening your upper back and relaxing your head forwards. Breathe deeply for another six breaths.

SYMPHYSIS PUBIS DISORDER (SPD)

Alleviate early stages of pubic pain by toning the deepest muscles of the pelvis linked to your pelvic floor muscles. Sit astride a chair facing backwards, feet solid on the floor. Press your sitting bones into the chair and breathe deeply as you extend your left arm up for four breaths. Repeat with your right arm.

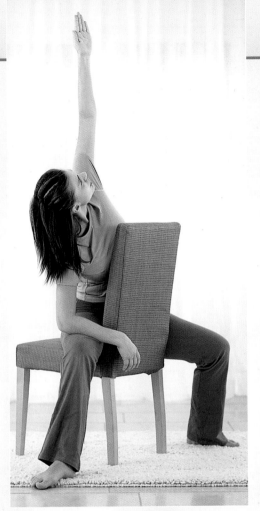

ANXIETY

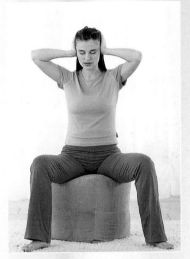

"Bee breath" helps to relieve mild depression and anxiety. Sit up straight with your hands over your ears and your eyes closed. Inhale deeply. Exhale slowly, making a buzzing sound that vibrates in your head. Repeat four times.

RELIEVING TENSION

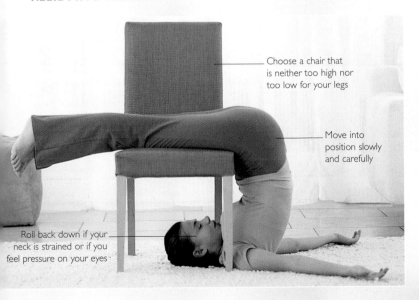

Choose a chair that is neither too high nor too low for your legs

Move into position slowly and carefully

Roll back down if your neck is strained or if you feel pressure on your eyes

If you can easily lift your legs over your head, use this supported Half plough pose to relax your brain and relieve tension and anxiety. Lie on the floor with your head under a chair and bring your legs over your head so that the tops of your thighs are supported by the chair seat. Support your shoulders with a folded blanket if your back needs to be lifted slightly. Rest your arms on the floor and relax for five to ten minutes, breathing evenly.

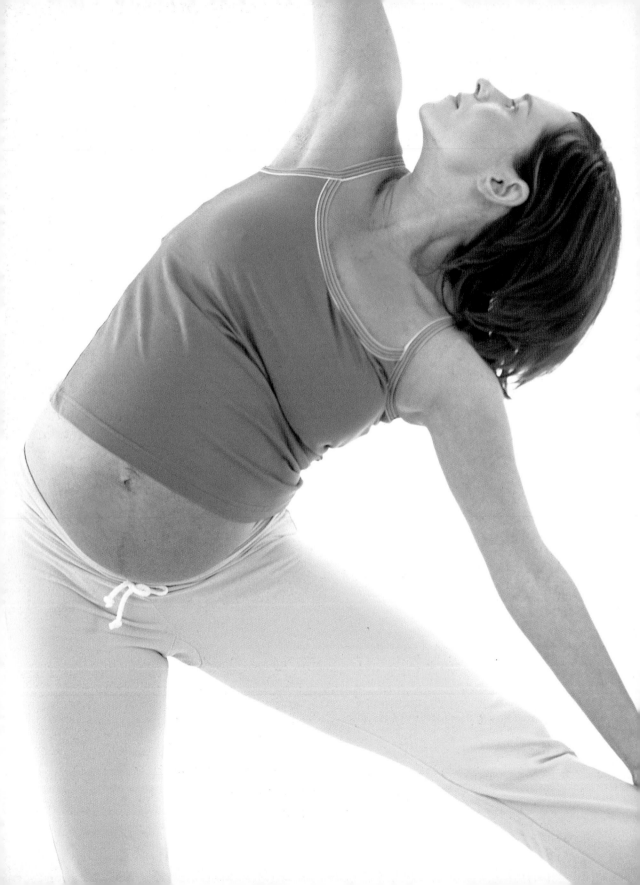

MID PREGNANCY

16 TO 34 WEEKS

This is the time to enjoy your pregnancy and your strong, vibrant and fit body. After much-needed rest and nurture in the early weeks, yoga can now energize and strengthen you to carry your growing baby with ease and confidence. Pregnancy is an adventure of self-transformation; a daily yoga practice, even if very short, followed by relaxation, creates the balance you need between permanence and all the changes in you and around you. Making friends with your baby through movement, touch, breath and sound is of the greatest importance. Fathers may welcome an invitation to take part in this exploration.

"Moon of the fifth month casts its shadow. The secret life stirs within me.
O my darling, I can hear your heartbeats"
Indian birth song

ALIGNMENT OF SPINE

Your growing abdomen inevitably affects the curvature of your spine, so it is important to maintain the correct posture. These standing exercises, based on Mountain pose, enable you to use rapid, easy checks to align your spine. The pelvic alignments of early pregnancy (pp.20–21) are also safe to do until thirty weeks, when the pressure of lying on your back may affect the blood flow to your baby.

> **CAUTIONS** Stand against a wall in front of a mirror when you align your spine for the first time so that you can check your alignment is indeed correct; often what "feels" right isn't actually so. If you have high blood pressure, skip step 2.

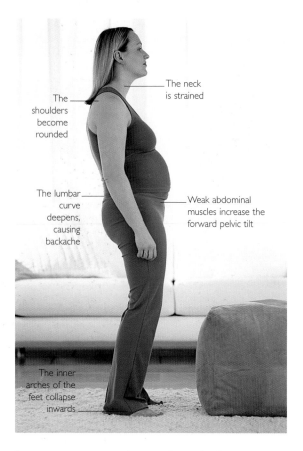

The neck is strained

The shoulders become rounded

The lumbar curve deepens, causing backache

Weak abdominal muscles increase the forward pelvic tilt

The inner arches of the feet collapse inwards

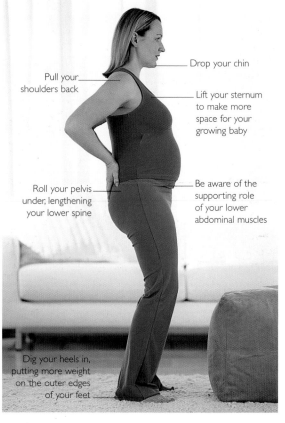

Drop your chin

Pull your shoulders back

Lift your sternum to make more space for your growing baby

Roll your pelvis under, lengthening your lower spine

Be aware of the supporting role of your lower abdominal muscles

Dig your heels in, putting more weight on the outer edges of your feet

Incorrect posture As your lower back caves in due to the growing weight of your baby, your neck extends forwards to compensate, creating an illusory sense of alignment. The greater weight bearing on the inner arches of your feet can cause you to waddle.

Correct posture Stand in Mountain pose with feet hip-width apart, knees slightly bent, and with your hands on your lower back to guide your pelvis into position. Breathe freely, aligning yourself along an inner axis from your crown, through your perineum, down to your feet.

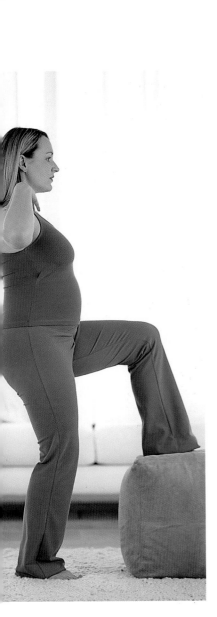

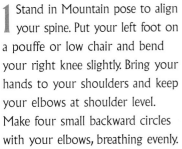

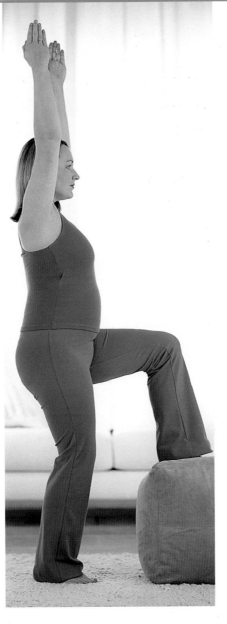

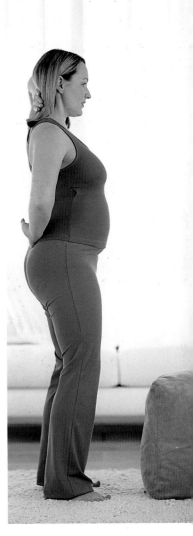

1 Stand in Mountain pose to align your spine. Put your left foot on a pouffe or low chair and bend your right knee slightly. Bring your hands to your shoulders and keep your elbows at shoulder level. Make four small backward circles with your elbows, breathing evenly.

2 Keep your head straight and raise your arms above your head, holding your fingers tight together. Drop your left hip and stretch your long back muscles. If you can remain comfortably in this pose, hold it for four breaths. Then repeat steps 1 and 2 on your right side.

3 For a quick alignment check, stand in Mountain pose and place one hand on the base of your neck and the other on your lumbar curve.

SUN SALUTATION
Surya Namaskar

Sun salutation stretches are invigorating, and infuse you with a positive outlook for the rest of the day. This sequence, adapted for pregnancy, tones your whole body without exertion in a short time and strengthens your cardiovascular and respiratory systems. You can pace yourself and modify the sequence to improve your stamina in a way that best suits your individual needs.

> **CAUTIONS**
> • If you are affected by SPD or groin pain, skip steps 7 and 10.
> • If you have recurrent sciatic pain, replace step 11 with the special application on page 93.
> • Practice on a non-slip surface.

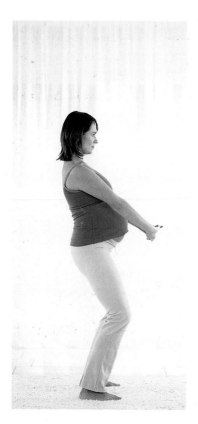

1 Stand in Mountain pose, feet hip-width apart and knees bent slightly. Exhale to centre yourself, interlock your fingers, turn your hands out and extend your arms.

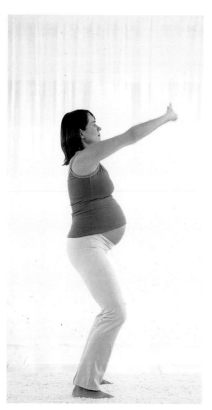

2 Take a deep in-breath and slowly raise your arms above your head without moving your lower body. Keep your head relaxed as you gaze straight ahead and remain grounded.

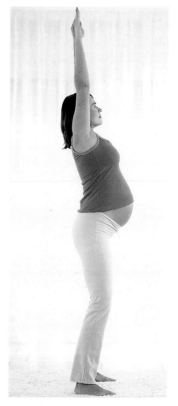

3 Unlock your fingers and face your palms forwards. Exhale and extend the stretch by pressing your heels down. Inhale and lift your rib cage.

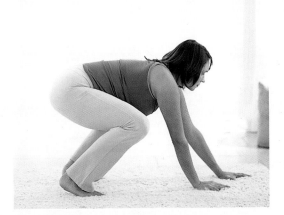

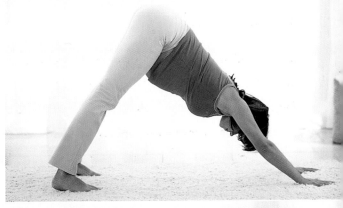

4 As you exhale, bend your knees, bring your arms down and walk your hands along the floor. If you can manage it, stretch your legs as you walk your hands forwards. *Alternatively, kneel down on all fours with your toes turned under.*

5 Inhale, straighten your legs and lift your sitting bones as high as possible in Dog pose. Keep your heels down if you can, or bend your knees. As you exhale, press your index fingers onto the floor to create a straight line from your wrists to your hips. Inhale again.

Adjust the angle of your knees to bring your buttocks as close to your feet as possible

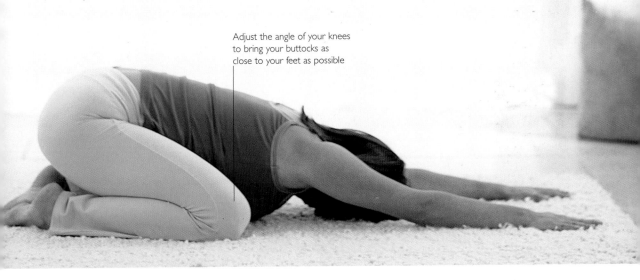

6 As you exhale, bend your knees, turning them out to allow for a comfortable forward stretch, and come down into Child's pose. Rest your forehead on the floor and relax for a couple of breaths. *End the Sun salutation sequence here if you feel tired or, if you are ready for more, continue with the rest of the sequence overleaf.*

WORK IN THE SEQUENCE

This Sun salutation sequence is achieved by breathing in and out continuously through the successive poses. It can also be performed more slowly by holding each pose, or resting, for several breaths. It is important that you maintain a steady rhythm, whether fast or slow, throughout the sequence.

▶

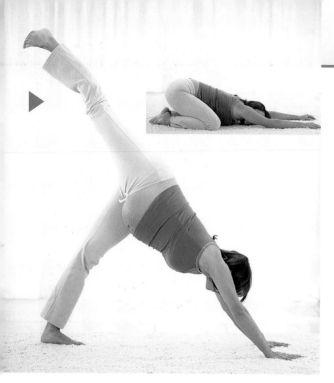

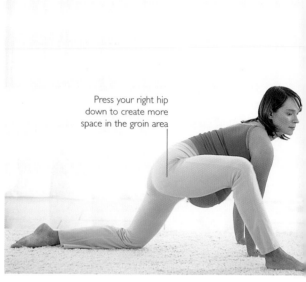

Press your right hip down to create more space in the groin area

7 From Child's pose, turn your toes under, inhale and lift into Dog pose. Form a strong base with your hands and feet, lift your right leg in the air and stretch into your heel as you exhale. Keep both knees bent if you find it easier. Then rest in Child's pose for a couple of deep breaths.

8 Inhale and shift your centre of gravity forwards so that as you kneel up on all fours, you can move your right leg and place your right foot on the floor outside your hands. As you exhale, push your right hip down to open your sacrum area and alleviate any discomfort created by your growing baby.

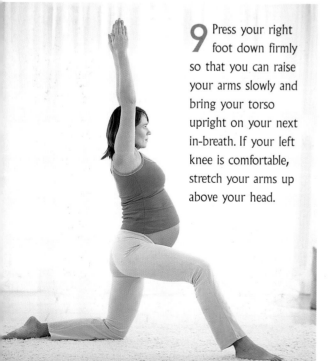

9 Press your right foot down firmly so that you can raise your arms slowly and bring your torso upright on your next in-breath. If your left knee is comfortable, stretch your arms up above your head.

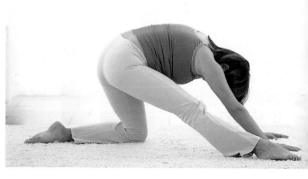

10 Exhale, straighten your right leg and lunge forwards to place your hands on the floor in line with your right foot. Relax your head. Rest in Child's pose, then repeat steps 7–10 with the left leg.

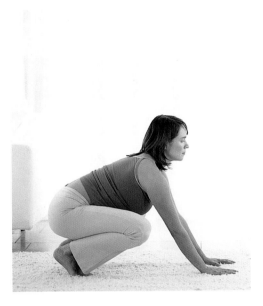

11 After resting in Child's pose, turn your toes under, take an in-breath and walk your hands back towards your body until you can roll back into a squat position. Keep your head aligned and push your heels down towards the floor to lengthen your spine.

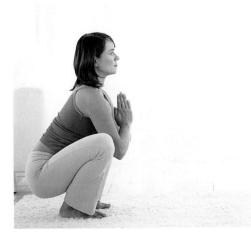

12 If you feel comfortable, hold the squat with your hands in Prayer pose and your elbows inside your knees for two breaths. Otherwise, use the momentum to stand up.

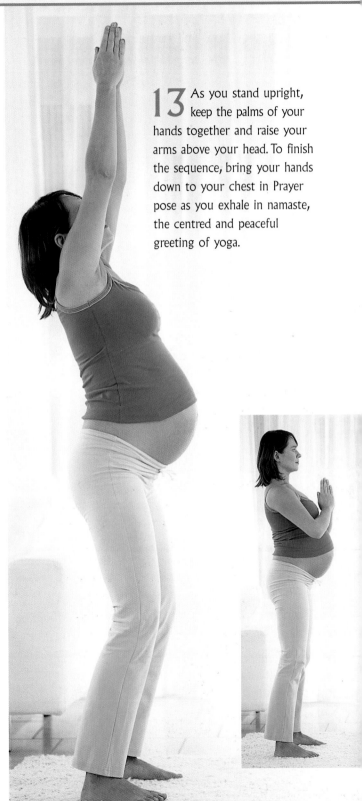

13 As you stand upright, keep the palms of your hands together and raise your arms above your head. To finish the sequence, bring your hands down to your chest in Prayer pose as you exhale in namaste, the centred and peaceful greeting of yoga.

STANDING TWISTS

These dynamic diagonal movements utilize all your torso muscles from the hips to the shoulders, taking pressure off your lower back. Such movements are most effective in building strength in the transverse abdominal muscles that support your fast-expanding uterus. According to your mood, alternate rhythmical swings with relaxed stretching from your lower spine up to your fingertips. Both will energize you in different ways, stimulating your breathing as well as your physical and mental coordination.

Look back at your heel to gain further stretch across the shoulders

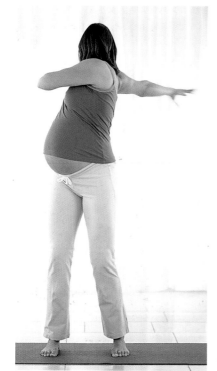

2 Move your feet further apart and extend the twist into a long standing stretch of your whole body. As you rotate to the right, raise your right arm up and extend your left arm down behind you. Feel the stretch through your body from your left heel to the fingertips of your left hand. Bend your knees before you rotate to the left and repeat the stretch on the other side.

1 Stand in Mountain pose with your knees slightly bent. Breathe freely and twist loosely from side to side, swinging your arms in turn across your body and back behind you.

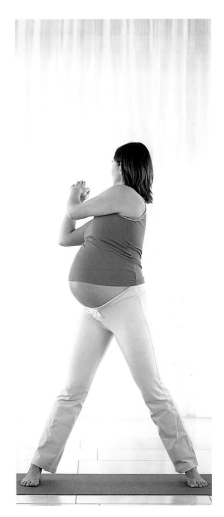

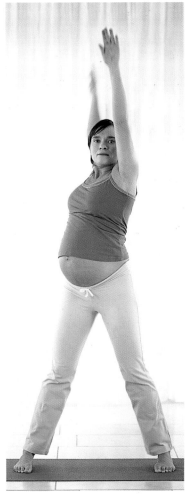

WORK IN THE POSE

There are many possible ways of breathing in these movements. As a rule, inhale on the upward stretches and exhale when you bend your knees to change sides. However, when you hold poses, you may wish to exhale in the stretch and then take a new breath before exhaling as you release out of the pose.

Bending your knees is essential for twisting your whole torso as opposed to just twisting your shoulders, which would result in weakening the lumbar spine during pregnancy.

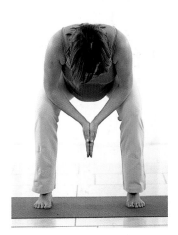

3 Stand firm with your feet wide apart and facing forwards. Press the palms of your hands together and twist your torso round to the right, pushing your right elbow back as you rotate both your shoulders. Breathe easily throughout, stretching further on each exhalation. Repeat alternately on each side four times.

4 Keep your feet facing forwards and twist your body round to the right while simultaneously raising your left arm out in front and your right arm behind you. Bend your knees and exhale as you lower your arms down and return to the centre. Repeat on the left side. Gradually lift your arms higher and higher in semi-circles of opposition until your hands meet above your head. Breathe energetically throughout.

5 As a counterpose, stand in a semi-squat with your feet parallel and your knees bent. Press your elbows onto your knees and relax your head down. If you wish, join your hands and point your fingers towards the floor.

EASY TRIANGLE TO MOON

These beautiful, classic poses give great value in stretching all the spinal muscles and helping you to create plenty more space inside for your growing baby. Use a chair as a support to ease the essential movements from your hips and rib cage. Even if you are an experienced practitioner of yoga, try this adapted sequence first for its benefits on your pregnant body.

CAUTIONS

• To avoid straining your neck, always move your head in line with your spine.
• Keep the hip bone of your standing leg well back to stretch the pelvic ligaments correctly.

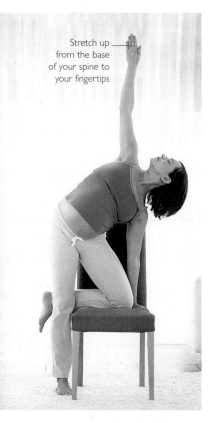

Stretch up from the base of your spine to your fingertips

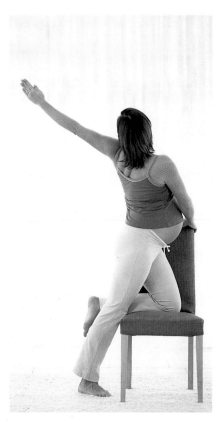

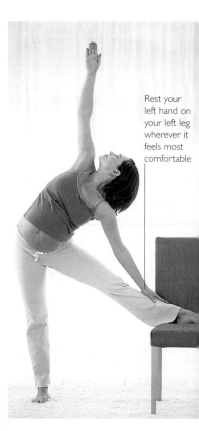

Rest your left hand on your left leg wherever it feels most comfortable

1 Stand on your right leg and rest your left knee on the chair seat. Raise your right arm, then gradually lower your left hand onto the chair seat without bending at the waist.

2 Without moving your legs, twist round to the left until you can comfortably hold the back of the chair with your right hand. Inhale and slowly extend your left arm back in line with your right shoulder. Breathe deeply.

3 Stand away from the chair so that as you extend your left leg, your foot is supported. Raise your right arm and stretch from the base of the spine. Exhale and turn your rib cage to the right.

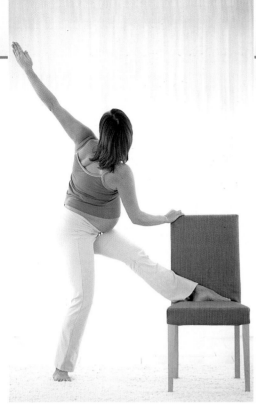

5 Place your left knee and arm on the chair seat and raise your right arm in this adapted Moon pose. Rest your upper body against the back of the chair and let your left knee and arm take most of your weight. Press your right rib cage and hip against the chair back to create more space in your body, and breathe deeply.

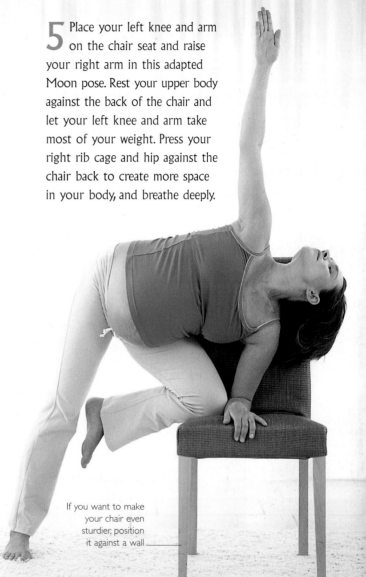

If you want to make your chair even sturdier, position it against a wall

4 Keeping your legs in the same position, twist to the left until you can rest your right hand on the back of the chair. Inhale and extend your left arm back with a deep rotation from the right hip. Bend your right knee to ease this movement. Without straining your neck, let your head follow the twist of your spine and look up at your left hand.

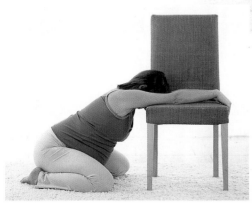

6 This wide kneeling position allows you to stretch with a straight back. Sit back on your heels in front of the chair with your knees wide apart. Rest your arms and forehead on the chair seat in a relaxed stretch. Take a few deep breaths and enjoy the open feeling generated by these poses. Repeat the whole sequence on the right side.

ADVANCED TRIANGLE TO MOON
Ardha Chandrasana

Classic standing poses such as these enable you to stretch gracefully upwards to the sky while using the pull of gravity to maintain a feeling of physical support and balance. Once your body is well grounded from your feet to your hips, you can extend your upper body sideways with a twisting movement of your whole spine in Triangle, and then enjoy a forgotten freedom in Moon pose.

BENEFITS These poses create a sense of space inside you. They also:
• Tone and pre-stretch the abdominal muscles, which continue to expand until your baby reaches his or her full size.
• Prevent and alleviate constipation.

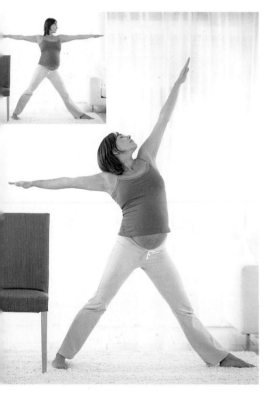

2 By bending over slowly to the left, you find yourself effortlessly in Triangle pose. Hold the pose for two breaths and then come up as slowly as you went down.

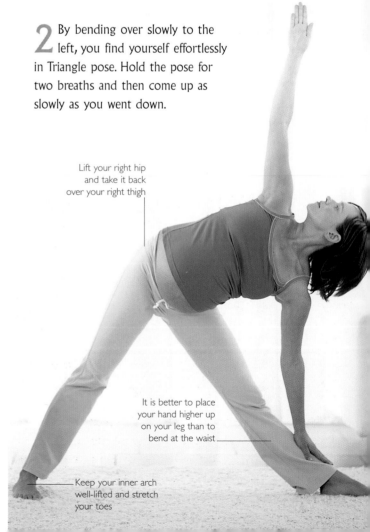

Lift your right hip and take it back over your right thigh

It is better to place your hand higher up on your leg than to bend at the waist

Keep your inner arch well-lifted and stretch your toes

1 Make a Triangle base by standing with your feet firmly apart. Turn your left foot out and extend your arms out at shoulder level in a relaxed stretch. Inhale, raise your left arm up, exhale and look at your left hand.

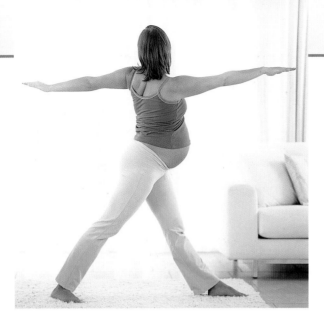

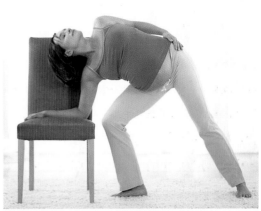

3 Without moving your legs or feet, breathe in and swing your extended arms round to the left. Press your right foot down and extend your left arm right back on an out-breath. Return slowly to the centre.

4 Stand to the left of the chair and make a stable Triangle base with your feet. Then bend your right knee and rest your right forearm on the chair seat. Turn your torso round to the left.

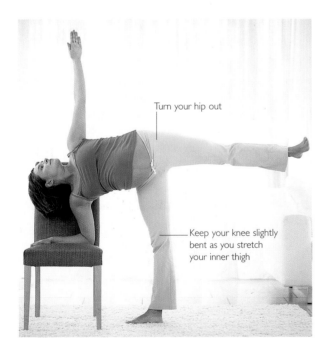

Turn your hip out

Keep your knee slightly bent as you stretch your inner thigh

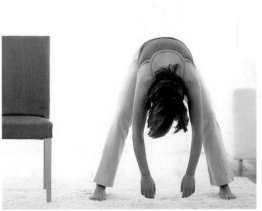

5 Extend your left leg out horizontally, keeping your centre of gravity above your right leg in your left hip. Rest your right shoulder against the chair back and raise your left arm above your head. Breathe deeply.

6 Rest in a loose Forward bend (p.27), relaxing your arms and head down. Keep your knees bent if this feels more comfortable. Breathe deeply. Repeat the sequence on the right side.

EASY ARCHER TO WARRIOR

These supported adaptations combine two classic yoga poses that develop the power, concentration and strength of a warrior; many cultures compare the courage required of mothers to that of warriors. In order to gain the full benefit from these robust poses without strain on the pelvic ligaments, use a chair to support your body and facilitate deep abdominal breathing.

CAUTIONS
• Use a sturdy chair for this pose. To make the chair as secure as possible, push it against a wall.
• Position yourself carefully at the edge of the chair seat. Make your back leg strong to give you stability.

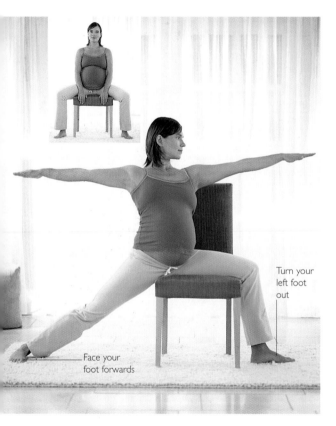

Turn your left foot out

Face your foot forwards

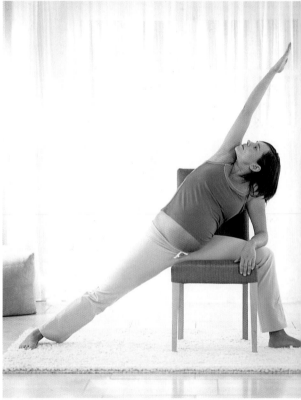

1 Sit tall on a chair with your knees wide apart and your feet at an angle that allows for maximum stability. Rest your hands on the chair seat and breathe deeply. Turn to your left and straighten your right leg. Extend your arms out at shoulder level and look at your left hand. Hold for three breaths.

2 Rest your left elbow on your left thigh and stretch your right arm up above your right ear to create a strong line from your right heel to your right hand. Turn your torso out as you stretch and breathe into your expanded right rib cage.

3 If you have enough energy for a supported Archer pose, keep your lower body in the same wide base and move your torso into an upright position. Pull back your right elbow at shoulder level as you stretch your left arm out in front of you. Hold for three breaths.

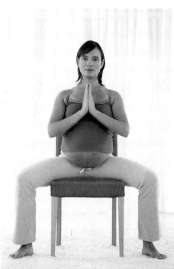

4 Bring your hands together in Prayer pose. Inhale, raise your arms above your head, push your elbows together and look up at your hands. Exhale in the stretch and focus your awareness on your back heel. Then lower your arms and bring your hands to your chest.

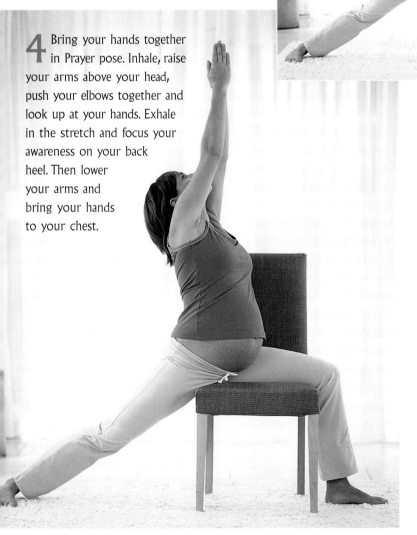

5 Sit squarely on the chair with your hands in Prayer pose. Take a few quiet breaths to ground yourself with your renewed strength. Be aware of your baby as you store this calm energy for the weeks ahead. Repeat steps 1–5 on the left side.

ADVANCED ARCHER TO WARRIOR
Virabhadrasana

In this dynamic sequence, energetic flowing movements develop naturally into classic held poses in order to gain maximum extension, freedom and precision, and a full enjoyment of your active body and mind. In just a few moments you can feel vital, light and strong, then return to your day with a renewed focus. When you reach Archer pose (step 5), set your intent with the imaginary arrow you send into the sky and energize yourself in the dynamic stillness.

BENEFITS AND CAUTIONS

This sequence strengthens you mentally and physically. Practise each step separately at first if you need to build up your stamina.

Do not attempt this sequence if you are affected by SPD or have pains in your lower abdomen.

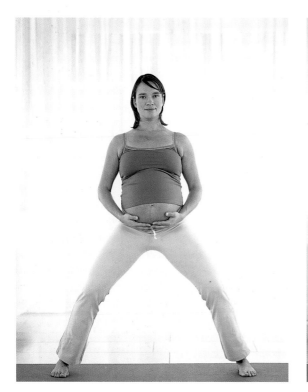

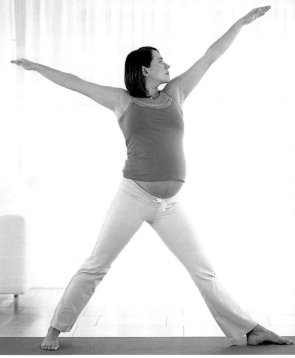

1 Stand with feet wide apart in Mountain pose. Bend your knees slightly and press down on your heels to align your spine. Release your chin down and place your hands under your abdomen. Breathe deeply, bending your knees more each time as you exhale.

2 Turn your left foot out. As you inhale, open your arms out and raise them up in a relaxed stretch above your shoulders until they form a wide V shape. Look up at your left hand. Exhale, bend your knees, lower your arms and turn your torso to the left.

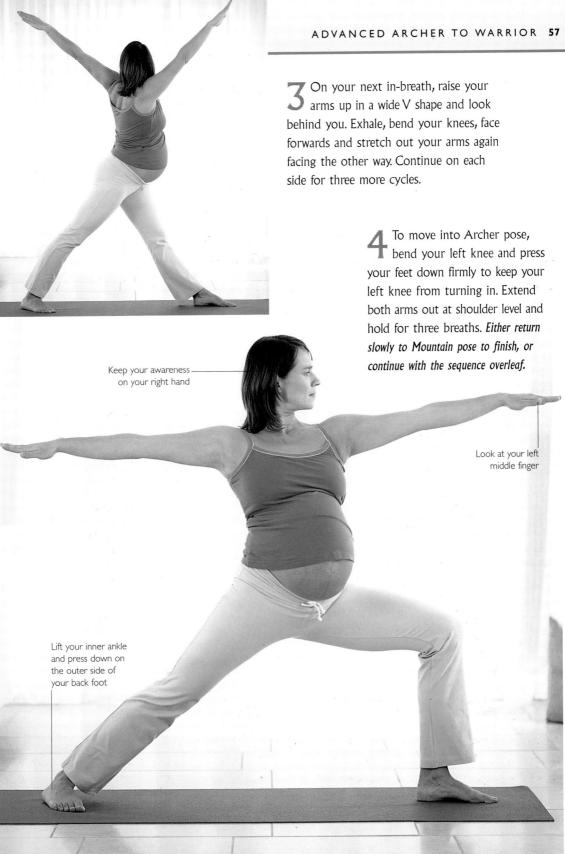

3 On your next in-breath, raise your arms up in a wide V shape and look behind you. Exhale, bend your knees, face forwards and stretch out your arms again facing the other way. Continue on each side for three more cycles.

4 To move into Archer pose, bend your left knee and press your feet down firmly to keep your left knee from turning in. Extend both arms out at shoulder level and hold for three breaths. *Either return slowly to Mountain pose to finish, or continue with the sequence overleaf.*

Keep your awareness on your right hand

Look at your left middle finger

Lift your inner ankle and press down on the outer side of your back foot

5 Continue to hold Archer pose as you bend your right arm, pull back your elbow and position your right hand by your shoulder. Inhale and raise your left arm to create a line parallel to that of your back leg.

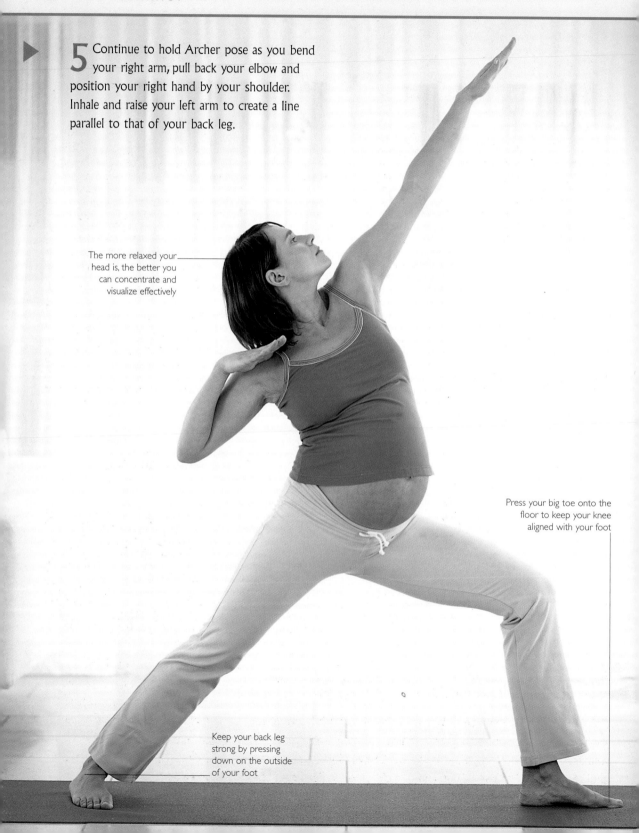

The more relaxed your head is, the better you can concentrate and visualize effectively

Press your big toe onto the floor to keep your knee aligned with your foot

Keep your back leg strong by pressing down on the outside of your foot

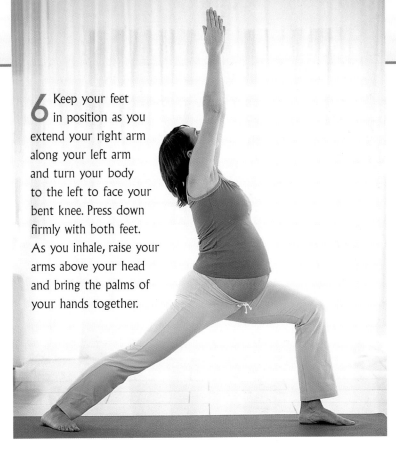

6 Keep your feet in position as you extend your right arm along your left arm and turn your body to the left to face your bent knee. Press down firmly with both feet. As you inhale, raise your arms above your head and bring the palms of your hands together.

WORK IN THE POSE

This sequence can be done in one energetic, flowing movement guided by the rhythm of your breathing. Alternatively, it can be done slowly: take your time to get in and out of each pose, returning to Mountain pose after each move to rest.

To avoid tension and increase relaxed stretching in these poses:
• Ensure that your shoulders and neck remain relaxed throughout.
• Always breathe abdominally.
• Check your centre of gravity in each pose.
• Remain aware of the connection between your core and extremities.
• Remember that your breathing animates your poses.

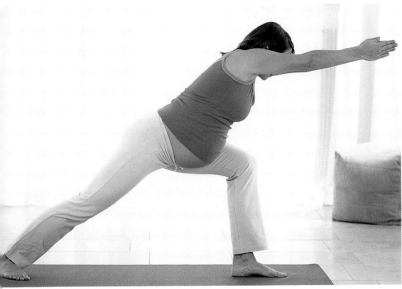

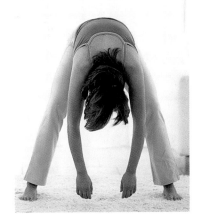

7 As you exhale, continue in Warrior pose with this forward lunge, which extends your whole spine in line with your back heel. Keep your feet in position and your hands joined. Slowly lower your arms until they are at shoulder height, and stretch for three deep breaths.

8 Relax your shoulders and neck in a standing Forward bend, letting your arms hang loosely. Bend your knees if this feels more comfortable. Return slowly to Mountain pose. Repeat the sequence on the right side.

TREE POSE
Vrksasana

Seek your balance from inside as you breathe in this beautiful pose. Whether you are new to yoga or not, follow this sequence to gain stability as you draw the muscles of your standing leg up to allow you to stretch upwards from the pelvis. Adjust your centre of gravity and spread your roots to expand in your space as your baby grows inside you.

> **CAUTIONS** Practise an easier pose with confidence rather than compromise your balance on the full pose. Avoid excessive pressure on the veins of your standing leg by holding the full pose for not more than 30 seconds while pregnant.

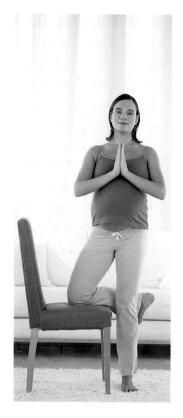

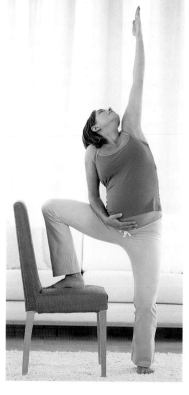

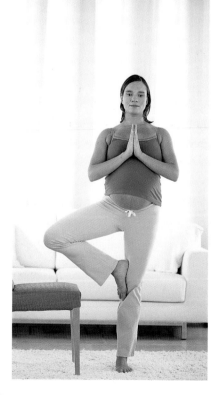

1 Rest your right knee on the seat of a chair, join your hands in Prayer pose and align your spine. Breathe freely.

2 Place your right foot on the chair to prepare for Tree pose and to deepen your abdominal breathing. Lift your left arm and stretch from heel to hand.

3 Exhale and press your right foot against your left leg, just above the inner knee. Join your hands in Prayer pose. Gaze ahead and breathe deeply to create balance from inside.

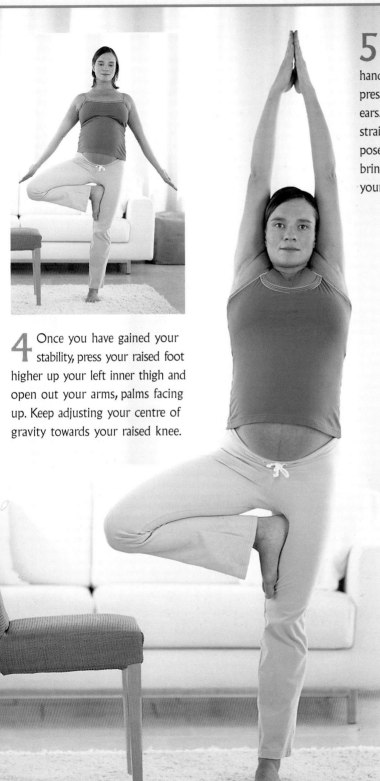

5 On an in-breath, raise your arms firmly above your head. Join your hands together in Prayer pose and press your upper arms against your ears. As you gain confidence, try to straighten your elbows. Hold Tree pose for three breaths, then slowly bring your arms down and release your raised leg.

4 Once you have gained your stability, press your raised foot higher up your left inner thigh and open out your arms, palms facing up. Keep adjusting your centre of gravity towards your raised knee.

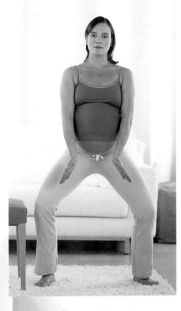

6 Return to a wide Mountain pose with your knees bent. Finish with an opening feminine mudra. Hold your joined hands, palms down, in front of your pubic bone. As you exhale, open your hands out along your thighs in an expanding inverted V shape. Repeat on the left side.

STANDING HIP OPENERS

Having strong, flexible pelvic joints is of special importance while you are pregnant. Movements such as these improve the circulation of the blood to all your organs, and particularly to your uterus. They also help you to move freely and comfortably in harmony with your new shape, and to gently increase your pelvic diameters to encourage your baby to move into a "head down" position.

> **CAUTION** If you are affected by SPD, avoid step 5. Practise steps 2, 3 and 6 using small, low-level circular knee movements instead. Hold step 4 for six breaths rather than three to strengthen the pelvic ligaments around the symphysis.

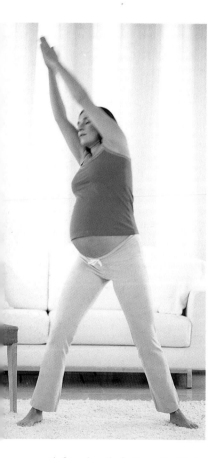

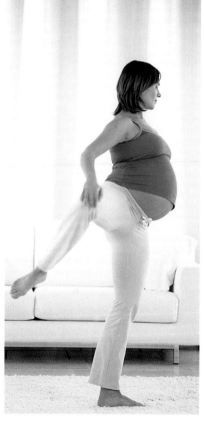

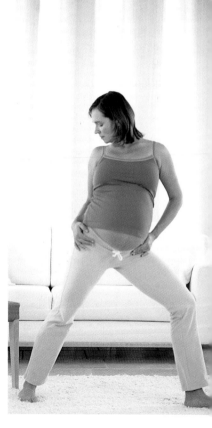

1 Stand with feet apart. Inhale, join your hands and lift your arms in a wide circle. Exhale and bend your knees as your arms drop. Repeat three times.

2 Stand tall with your feet hip-width apart. On an in-breath, bend your right leg and lift your knee high. Hold your knee up with your right hand if this helps.

3 Exhale, gently land your right foot on the floor behind you and rotate your torso to the right. Bring your leg back. Repeat steps 2 and 3 three times on each side.

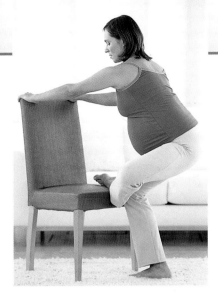

Open up a welcoming space for your baby with this uplifting, life-affirming movement

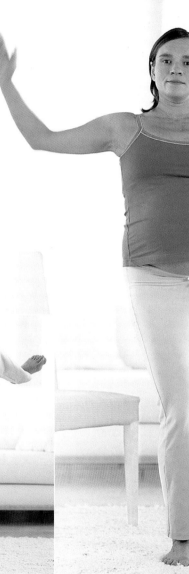

4 As a counterpose, stand in front of a sturdy chair, hold onto the chair back and bend your knees. Lift your left leg and place your left foot, sole facing up, on the seat. Gently pull your left hip down for three deep breaths. Repeat on the other side.

5 To create more space in your pelvis, stand facing the chair with your knees slightly bent. Rest your forearms on the seat and hold onto the chair back. Lift your bent left leg behind you, opening your hip out, and release gently. Repeat three times on each side.

6 End this sequence by circling both hands in the air, accompanied a dynamic circling of each knee out to the side. You may even begin to take off with a tiny jump, so jump for joy, whatever your mood.

STRONG CENTRING POSES

These dynamic stretches, which are rooted in the ancient eastern links between yoga and martial arts, actively prepare your body and mind for labour. The more you can mobilize your inner strength now, the better you will be able to relax and surrender later when needed without letting your energy levels dip. The flow of your breath brings together the physical, mental and emotional aspects of yourself and helps you to centre using strong contrasts of extension and release, contraction and relaxation.

CAUTIONS Begin with your knees slightly bent and only progress to semi-squats if you are unaffected by SPD or groin pains:
• Don't hold semi-squats or squats.
• If you have difficulty coming out of a pose, drop forwards onto all fours or onto a stool, rest, and then stand up. Lean against a wall if you require support for your back.

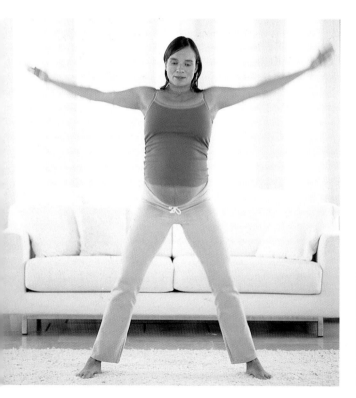

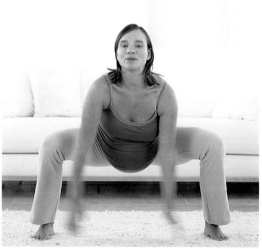

1 Stand in Mountain pose with your feet wide apart and arms extended out at shoulder level. Exhale, drop your arms and bend your knees in a semi-squat. Inhale, lift your arms and straighten your legs. Repeat three times.

2 Lower down into a wide squat, or semi-squat, as you exhale. Bring your hands together in a gathering gesture and, as you inhale, stand up and open your arms out in a wide circle above your head. Exhale down again and repeat three times.

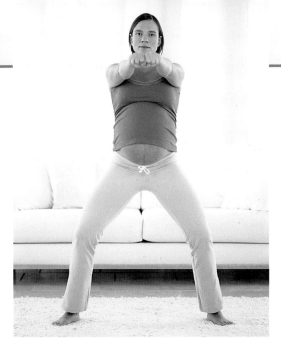

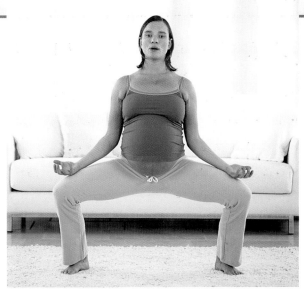

3 Stand strong with feet apart and knees bent. Extend your hands out at shoulder level, palms down, and make fists. Take a deep breath and hold it as long as you can while tightening your fists.

4 Exhale with a deep "Aaah" sound as you drop into a semi-squat position. Keep your back upright and aligned as you drop down. Gently release your arms and rest your hands, palms facing up, on your knees.

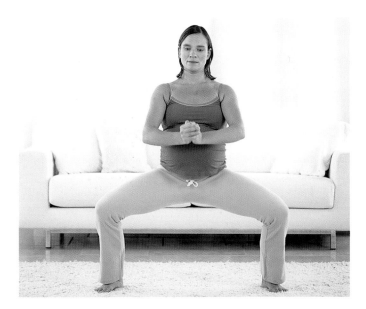

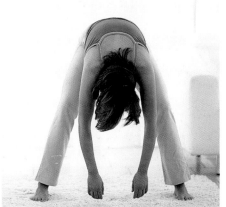

5 Stand strong with feet wide apart and knees bent. Make a fist with one hand at chest height and wrap the other hand around it. Inhale and raise your hands to face level. Exhale and bend your knees. Come back up slowly on the next in-breath. Repeat three times, aligning yourself with your out-breath.

6 Rest in a standing Forward bend, relaxing your arms and head down loosely. Keep your knees bent if this feels more comfortable. Breathe freely, relaxing your shoulders and neck fully.

EASY KNEELING STRETCHES

Kneeling on the floor while pregnant is often more comfortable than sitting. It is also a traditional birthing position, which midwives now encourage in many maternity hospitals. Kneeling stretches have special value in stretching your pelvic muscles together with your lower back and buttock muscles. These first easy stretches utilize your birthing muscles in ways that may not be familiar to you, even if you are experienced with yoga. They are best performed slowly in a relaxed way.

ONE-FOOT PIGEON POSE Eka pada Rajakapotasana

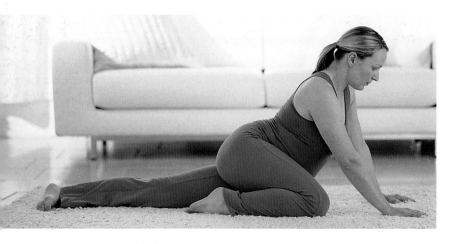

1 Kneel comfortably and place your hands on the floor in front of you. Keep your arms straight so that your spine is well aligned. Extend your left leg out behind you and turn your foot in, letting your hip drop. Hold for four deep breaths, then release.

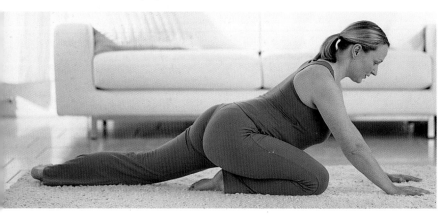

2 Turn your left foot out and feel your hip pulling up as you stretch into your left heel. Keep your neck soft and in line with your spine. Hold for four deep breaths. Slowly bring your leg forwards into a kneeling position. Repeat steps 1 and 2 with your right leg.

PIGEON POSE EXTENSION

Kneel with your hands on the floor in front of you. Slide your left foot across your body so that it rests comfortably under your groin. Extend your right leg out behind you. Once you are aligned in this pose, raise your left arm and stretch from your right toes to the tips of your left fingers. Hold for four breaths. Change sides and repeat with the other leg.

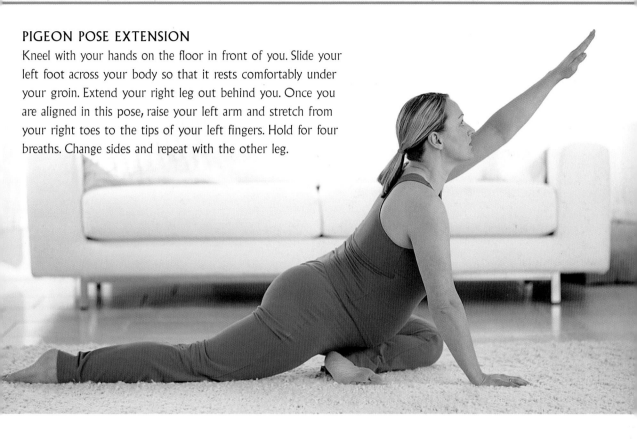

FLOOR EXTENSION

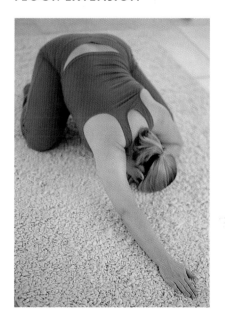

Position yourself in Cat pose: sit back on your heels with your arms bent and rest your forehead either on the floor, on your hands or on a cushion. Avoid lifting your buttocks as you stretch your left arm out in front of you. Hold for four breaths, elongating your spine with each out-breath. Repeat with the right arm.

RESTING POSE

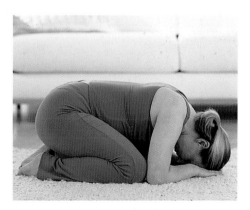

Rest in Cat pose with your knees out at a comfortable angle. Enjoy the safe "den" created by your joined knees, elbows and forehead. Breathe deeply into the spaces created in your groin area and upper back.

DYNAMIC KNEELING STRETCHES

In these stretches, balancing on one hand and one knee provides the base for full body extensions. Use these poses if you work at a desk or have been sitting down for a while, or after a car journey. They will help to create more growing space for your baby during those times when you wonder how any further growth is possible. If you are new to yoga, the careful positioning required in these stretches will help you to develop your sense of balance.

> **BENEFITS** Kneeling stretches can:
> • Prevent stretch marks appearing or help to control them.
> • Help stretch any existing scar tissue in the abdomen.
> • Offer a positive response when you feel that your pregnancy is overwhelming you.

SIMPLE DIAGONAL STRETCH

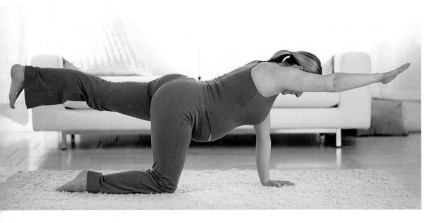

1 Start on all fours on the floor with your hands positioned beneath your shoulders. When you feel stable, inhale and extend your right arm and left leg out straight. Keep your middle back level like a table top and look down as you exhale in the stretch.

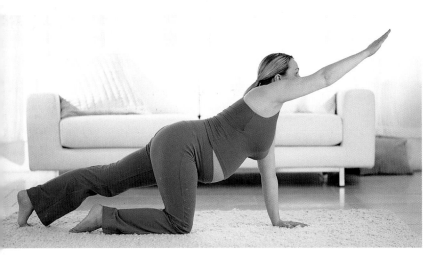

2 On your next in-breath, lower your left foot to the floor and raise your right arm up by your ear. Hold the stretch in a strong line from foot to hand for three deep abdominal breaths. Rest if needed *(see right)*. Then repeat steps 1 and 2 with your right leg and left arm.

TWISTING STRETCH

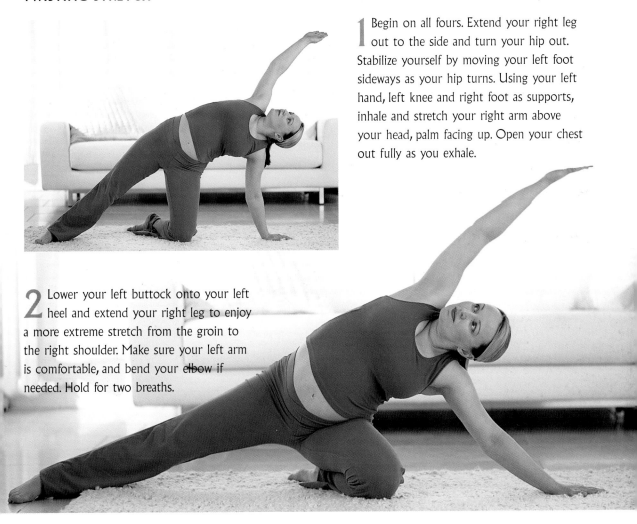

1 Begin on all fours. Extend your right leg out to the side and turn your hip out. Stabilize yourself by moving your left foot sideways as your hip turns. Using your left hand, left knee and right foot as supports, inhale and stretch your right arm above your head, palm facing up. Open your chest out fully as you exhale.

2 Lower your left buttock onto your left heel and extend your right leg to enjoy a more extreme stretch from the groin to the right shoulder. Make sure your left arm is comfortable, and bend your elbow if needed. Hold for two breaths.

RESTING POSE

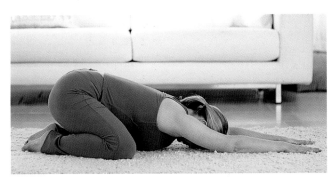

Complete this sequence with an extended Cat pose. Open your knees to a comfortable width, rest your arms on the floor in front of you and hold the pose for six deep breaths.

ADVANCED KNEELING STRETCHES
Virabhadrasana / Ardha Chandrasana

Let the flow of your breathing lead you through a succession of classic yoga poses that provide a dynamic yet safe workout of your whole body in just a few minutes. Starting and finishing with a feeling of inner peace and awareness of your baby is most important. If you are experienced at yoga, these poses will put your strength, flexibility and balance to good use once you are warmed up.

BENEFITS These stretches are well suited for an evening practice: kneeling protects the symphysis pubis while enabling you to gain all the benefits from standing poses. Steps 1 and 2, and 3 and 4, can be split into two separate sequences.

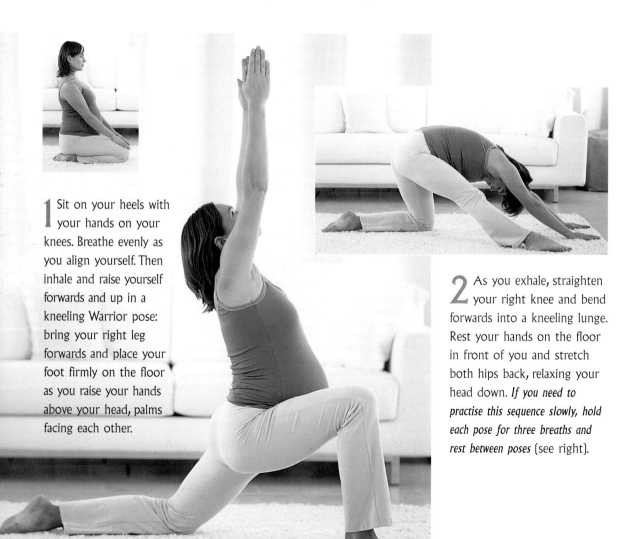

1 Sit on your heels with your hands on your knees. Breathe evenly as you align yourself. Then inhale and raise yourself forwards and up in a kneeling Warrior pose: bring your right leg forwards and place your foot firmly on the floor as you raise your hands above your head, palms facing each other.

2 As you exhale, straighten your right knee and bend forwards into a kneeling lunge. Rest your hands on the floor in front of you and stretch both hips back, relaxing your head down. *If you need to practise this sequence slowly, hold each pose for three breaths and rest between poses* (see right).

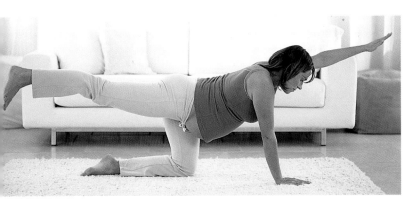

3 On your next in-breath, bend your right knee and move your centre of gravity forwards so that you balance on your right hand and left knee. Extend your left arm forwards and your right leg back in a strong horizontal line from heel to fingertips. Exhale in this stretch.

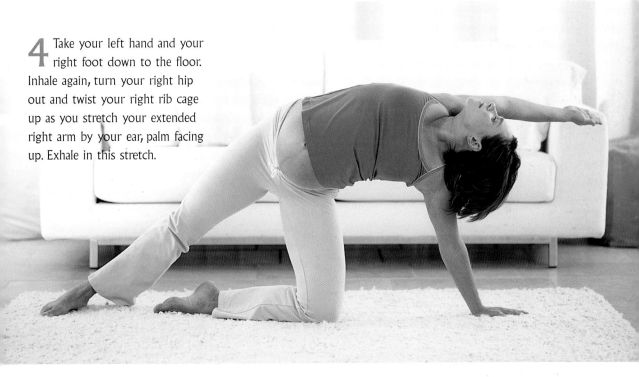

4 Take your left hand and your right foot down to the floor. Inhale again, turn your right hip out and twist your right rib cage up as you stretch your extended right arm by your ear, palm facing up. Exhale in this stretch.

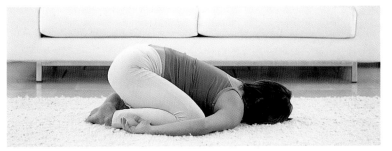

5 Slowly return to a kneeling position with the next flow of breath. Rest in Turtle pose, folding your arms back around your legs and resting the side of your head on the floor. *If you can relax in this pose, hold for three breaths or more, otherwise relax in Cat pose* (p.67).

SITTING CHAIR STRETCHES

Sitting on a chair to stretch enables you to receive all the benefits of seated yoga postures in an easy, comfortable position, right up to labour. The two mini workouts shown here can be done at odd moments through your day whenever you have time for a small break. Within a few minutes, these grounded spinal stretches will enliven you and involve you actively with your growing baby: such focused breathing, stretching and affirmative postures create a positive mode of interaction with your baby long before birth. Try to practise the stretches daily so that you can bond with your baby and look forwards to becoming a mother.

BENEFITS These adapted sitting poses have no counter-indications and benefit all pregnant women by:
• Increasing the flexibility of the lower spine and hips without risk of over-stretching pelvic ligaments.
• Promoting focused, deeper abdominal breathing.
• Stretching and relaxing the shoulder muscles.
• Aiding the mental and physical transition to motherhood during a busy time of life.

SEATED HIP ROLLS

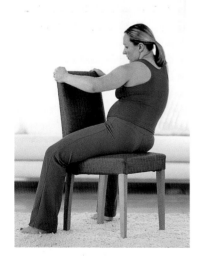

Sit astride a chair facing backwards. Hold onto the back of the chair with both hands and roll your hips in slow motion, pressing alternately on each sitting bone. Breathing evenly, roll clockwise in a circle, then anti-clockwise, several times.

SEATED TWISTS

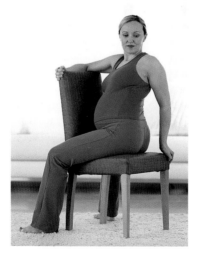

Place your left hand on the chair seat behind your back and use your right forearm and hand as a fulcrum to gently twist your whole torso round to the left. Breathe deeply, then repeat on the right side.

SEATED SUN WHEEL

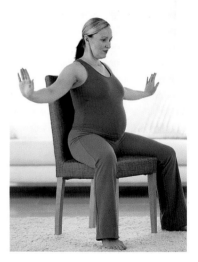

Sit upright on the chair with your legs apart. Push your hands out to either side as you exhale. Stretch into your wrists. Draw your hands back in as you inhale, then push them out again on the next out-breath. Practise again slowly.

SEATED FORWARD BEND SEQUENCE

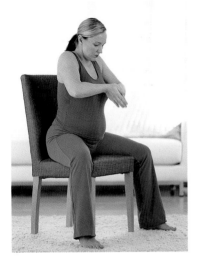

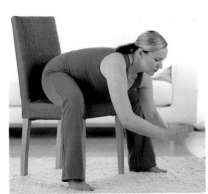

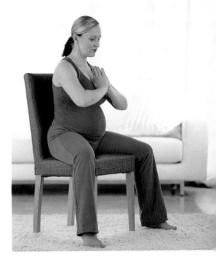

1 Join your hands in Prayer pose at chest height, fingers pointing down. Relax your shoulders and neck. Take a deep in-breath.

2 As you exhale, lunge forwards and lower your arms towards the floor. Inhale and draw your hands out and up in a circular movement.

3 Return your hands to chest height as you exhale to complete the movement. Breathe deeply, focusing inwards. Close your eyes if you wish.

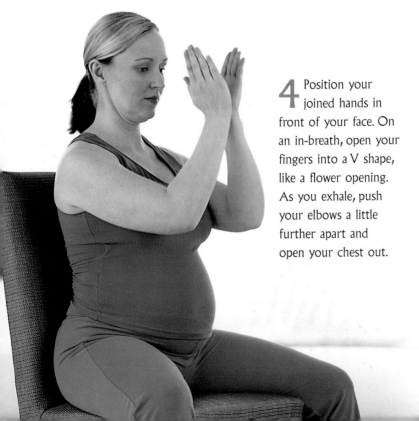

4 Position your joined hands in front of your face. On an in-breath, open your fingers into a V shape, like a flower opening. As you exhale, push your elbows a little further apart and open your chest out.

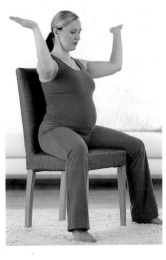

5 Move your hands, with palms face up, and elbows apart to open your chest. Then release and relax your arms.

SITTING STRETCHES

Suppleness in the hips can make childbirth easier. It is especially good to work on the hip joints while in a seated position, as the floor takes the weight of your body, allowing you to relax your hips and move freely. In this sequence, using a cushion under your bent knee makes the stretches safe and comfortable. From this steady base you can work with each out-breath to tone and elongate your spinal muscles through relaxed arm extensions. Focus on keeping your lower body planted on the floor as you stretch.

BENEFITS These poses aim to:
• Create space under the rib cage for your baby to expand into.
• Ease pressure caused by your baby's kicks or head.
• Encourage your baby to move into a central "head down" position.
• Tone the thoracic muscles supporting the breasts.
• Tone the abdominal muscles.

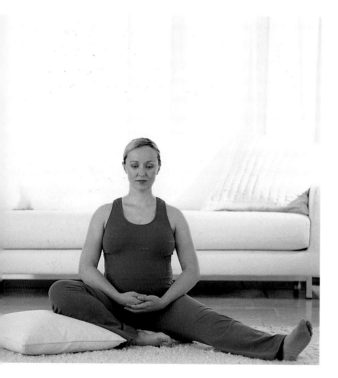

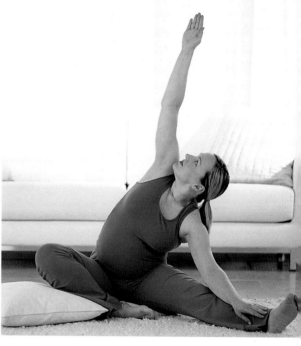

1 Sit on the floor with your legs as wide apart as feels comfortable. Bend your right knee so that your foot is close to your groin, with the sole of your foot against your left inner thigh. Use a cushion to support your bent knee comfortably. Rest your hands on your abdomen and breathe evenly, sitting up tall.

2 Stretch your left arm along your extended left leg. At the same time, turn your right shoulder back as if trying to look behind you. Inhale, stretch your right arm above your head and look up at your hand. Stretch deeper as you exhale, keeping your shoulders and neck relaxed.

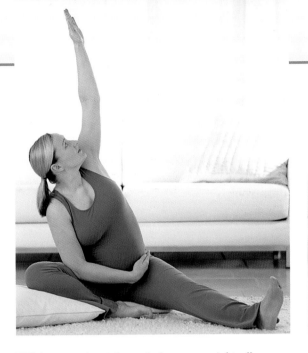

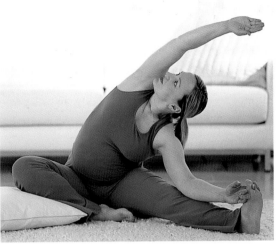

3 Lean to the right and place your right elbow on your right thigh, as close to your knee as you can. Rest your arm loosely across your abdomen. Turn your left shoulder back, twisting your spine upwards from its base. Inhale and stretch up with your left hand.

4 Exhale, swing your body to the left and hook your big toe with your index finger. If you can't reach your toe, use a yoga belt around your foot. Use your left elbow as a fulcrum to turn your torso out as you inhale and extend your right arm over your head.

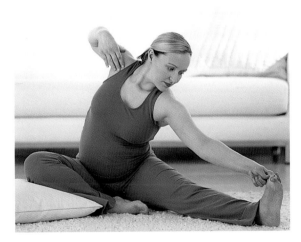

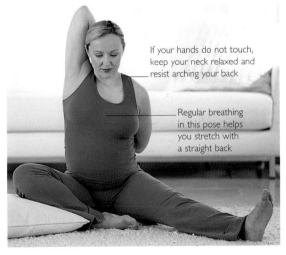

If your hands do not touch, keep your neck relaxed and resist arching your back

Regular breathing in this pose helps you stretch with a straight back

5 Still holding your big toe – or with the back of your hand against your inner leg wherever it feels most comfortable – bend your right elbow and stretch it back in line with your left arm, as if pulling back a powerful bow. Breathe deeply, stretch into your left heel, and press your right knee down.

6 Return to the centre. Inhale, extend your right arm up, exhale, bend your elbow and let your forearm drop behind your back. Inhale and bend your left arm behind your back. If your fingers meet, hook them together to stretch further as you exhale. Repeat the sequence on the other side.

WIDE-OPEN STRETCHES
Upavista Konasana

In this dynamic set of sitting poses, your legs are wide apart and your hips are open. This wide base is an efficient way to stretch out and strengthen the upper body while bringing increasing mobility to the lower back and hips. This sequence can be exhilarating if you feel energetic, but it can also energize you if you are tired. All these poses – practised either as a sequence or separately – will give you power from your base so close to the ground.

> **CAUTIONS**
> • To protect your lower back, you must sit up straight in this pose.
> • If you are a dancer or an experienced yogini, or your joints are very loose, be careful to avoid over-stretching in these poses. Don't stretch your legs wider than 120°.

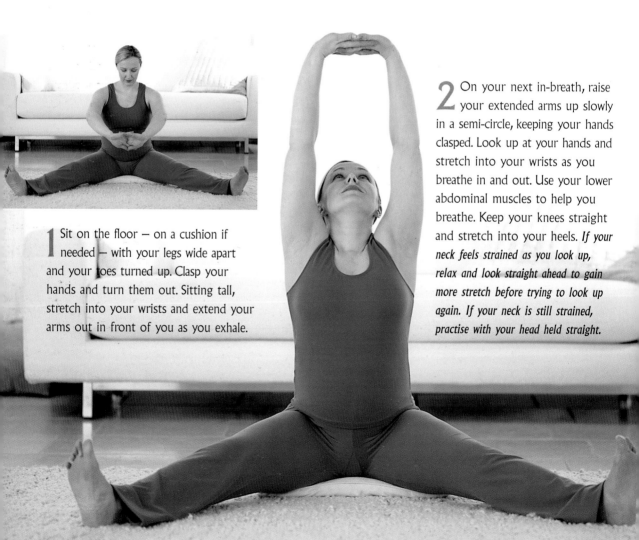

1 Sit on the floor – on a cushion if needed – with your legs wide apart and your toes turned up. Clasp your hands and turn them out. Sitting tall, stretch into your wrists and extend your arms out in front of you as you exhale.

2 On your next in-breath, raise your extended arms up slowly in a semi-circle, keeping your hands clasped. Look up at your hands and stretch into your wrists as you breathe in and out. Use your lower abdominal muscles to help you breathe. Keep your knees straight and stretch into your heels. *If your neck feels strained as you look up, relax and look straight ahead to gain more stretch before trying to look up again. If your neck is still strained, practise with your head held straight.*

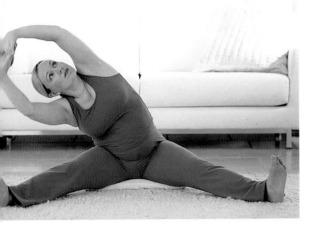

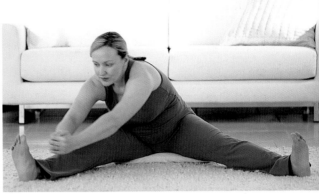

3 As you exhale, lean over to the right as far as you can towards your right leg, pressing into your wrists. Turn the muscles of your left leg out to maintain a strong, wide base. Repeat on the left side. *If you are ready for more, stretch in a continuous circular motion from right to left.*

4 Sit with your legs wide apart, toes turned up and your hands clasped as if grasping a huge stick. Inhale deeply and stretch your hands towards your right foot. Exhale and draw your hands round to your left foot, then to your waist and back to your right foot as if stirring a large pot. Reverse sides and repeat.

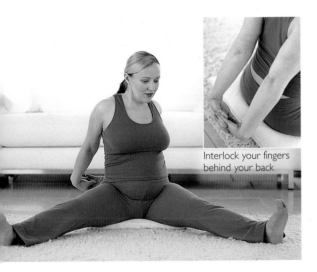

Interlock your fingers behind your back

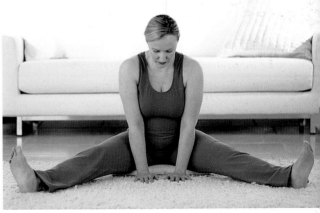

5 Sitting tall with your legs wide apart, extend your arms behind your back and interlock your fingers. Stretch into your wrists, pulling your shoulders back. Hold for three deep breaths using your lower abdominal muscles.

6 Unclasp your hands and position them on the floor just in front of you so that you can lift your upper body on an in-breath and use your abdominal and back muscles on the out-breath. This pose connects you with the effective yet gentle power of your birthing muscles.

FROM SITTING TO STANDING

Just as your balance and centre of gravity are affected by the increasing weight of your baby, so changing position requires more attention. This sequence enables you to keep your centre of gravity in the pelvis, protect your spine, and – once upright – enjoy a feeling of lightness and perfect alignment. Thus, by adapting the principles of yoga, this simple, necessary process of getting up from the floor is transformed into a positive, harmonious stretch that you will also find invaluable later on when playing with your baby.

> **CAUTIONS** Breathe fully as you move and always come up on an in-breath. Make use of supports to protect your knees and back, and check that your weight is evenly balanced. Even if you can squat easily, it is now recommended that women avoid holding unsupported squatting positions while they are pregnant.

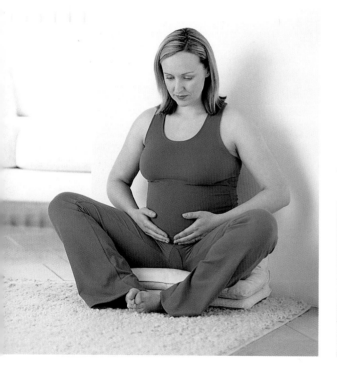

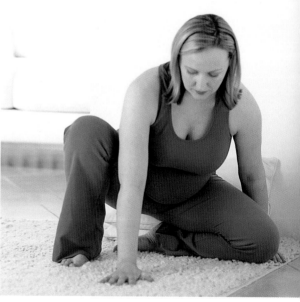

1 Times when you can sit quietly and be aware of your baby are precious bonding opportunities. Sit in classic Butterfly pose *(p.21)* with the soles of your feet joined. Place your hands on your abdomen and massage your baby with whatever strokes feel good. Shed your preoccupations with each out-breath.

2 From sitting, slide your left foot in close to your body. Plant your right foot on the floor in front of you. Inhale and lift your weight onto your hands. Slide your buttocks forwards to rest on your left heel as you exhale. *Repeat this movement slowly for an effective stretch of the muscles in your lower back and groin area.*

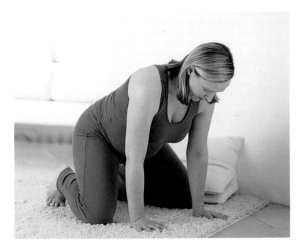

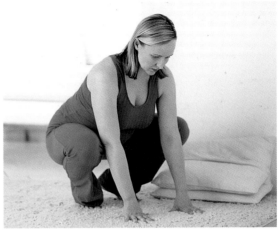

3 Move your left hand forwards and place your right knee on the floor so that you come onto all fours. Ideally, your knees should be in line with your hands and your feet in line with your knees. Move your weight slowly back towards your heels.

4 Continue to move back until your knees lift up off the floor. Then walk your hands backwards until you find yourself on tiptoes in a squatting position with your knees outside your arms. *Repeat again slowly if you want to stretch your lower back muscles.*

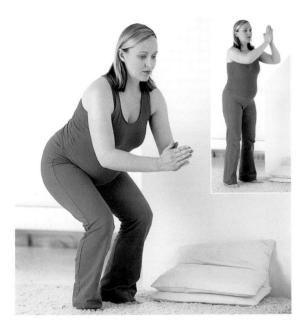

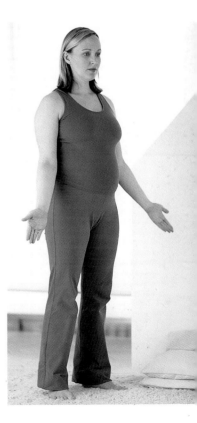

6 As you stand in a fully upright position, keep your hands in Prayer pose and extend your arms above your head for a complete stretch. Then bring your arms down to your sides with the palms of your hands opened out. *You may wish to repeat this hand movement with the affirmation, I am open and ready.*

5 With your hands so close to your body, your weight naturally will tip back. Inhale deeply, join your hands in Prayer pose and press your feet down as you slowly uncurl your spine to stand upright.

PELVIC FLOOR STRETCHES

The interwoven muscles that link the base of your spine with the front of your pelvis are most important. Their strength and elasticity contribute to a sound posture, the healthy functioning of organs in the lower abdomen and to how your vagina is transformed into a birth canal and reverts to its optimal tone after the birth. Gaining awareness and control of these muscles through breathing is vital; the earlier you start these exercises, the better. Frequent short practices for a few minutes daily in a relaxed atmosphere are most effective.

> **BENEFITS** These yoga stretches with deep breathing help you to:
> • Feel in control of your body and reduce any anxieties you might have about giving birth.
> • Enhance your sex life.
> • Give birth to your baby without distress by relying on the power of your breathing.
> • Prevent or relieve haemorrhoids.

PELVIC FLOOR INNER STRETCH

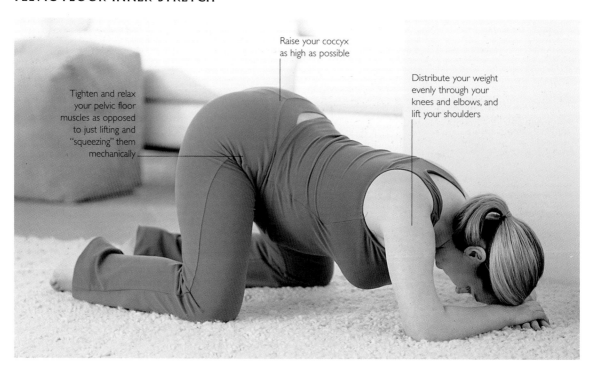

Raise your coccyx as high as possible

Tighten and relax your pelvic floor muscles as opposed to just lifting and "squeezing" them mechanically

Distribute your weight evenly through your knees and elbows, and lift your shoulders

Kneel in Cat pose with your knees wide apart. Lean forwards on your elbows and rest your head on your hands. Inhale and tighten your anal sphincter first. Release it fully on an out-breath. Repeat three times. Now focus on your urethra, which is key to bladder control. Tighten and release it in quick succession as you breathe evenly. Finally, focus on the muscles on each side of the vagina: draw these muscles inwards as much as you can. Release them slowly with a long exhalation, relaxing all your pelvic muscles. Repeat several times.

SEATED PELVIC FLOOR STRETCH

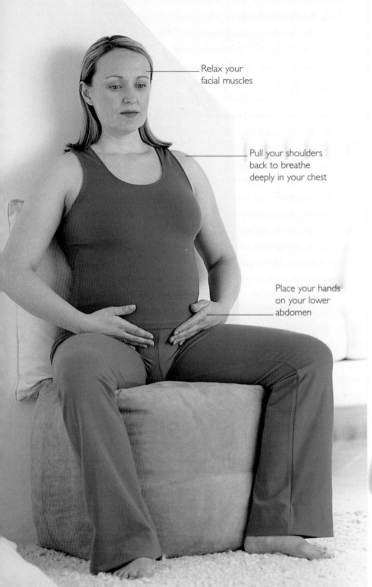

Relax your
facial muscles

Pull your shoulders
back to breathe
deeply in your chest

Place your hands
on your lower
abdomen

PELVIC FLOOR MUSCLES

The hammock of muscles lying at the base of
your torso supports the uterus, bowel and
bladder, and serves to close the entrances
to the vagina, rectum and urethra. During
pregnancy, an increase in progesterone causes
the pelvic floor muscles to soften and relax.

CROSS SECTION AT 32 WEEKS

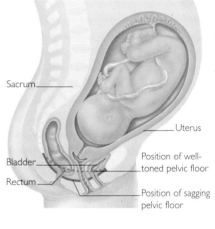

Sacrum

Uterus

Bladder

Position of well-
toned pelvic floor

Rectum

Position of sagging
pelvic floor

THE PERINEUM

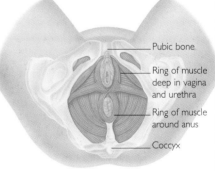

Pubic bone

Ring of muscle
deep in vagina
and urethra

Ring of muscle
around anus

Coccyx

Sit upright on a pouffe or chair with your knees apart.
Ensure that your spine is well supported, so use a
spare cushion if needed. Place your hands on your
lower abdomen, just under your baby. Focus on your
pelvic floor muscles by tightening and releasing them.

Then as you breathe in, draw them in and up as high
as you can using your lower back and abdominal
muscles. At the end of your in-breath, release your
pelvic floor very slowly as you exhale, lengthening
your exhalation as much as you can.

BREATH & AWARENESS

By placing your hands on different parts of your body while you breathe in and out, you can gain increasing awareness of your breathing as a tool that connects you physically, emotionally and spiritually with your body and your baby. This action also involves your involuntary muscles, enabling you to increase your breathing capacity, promote good muscle tone with all its associated benefits and make better use of your breathing to alter your mood. Mudras, with their opening and closing movements, provide a symbolic focus for this combined activity of breath, awareness and relaxation.

BENEFITS Section breathing in pregnancy helps you to:
• Respond to added pressures and constraints by expanding your breathing capacity. Practise twice a day if you are expecting two or more babies.
• Involve your pelvic muscles in the flow of each breath. For maximum benefit, tilt your pelvis back slightly while your lower back is supported.

SECTION BREATHING

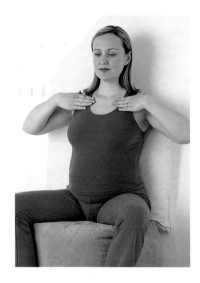

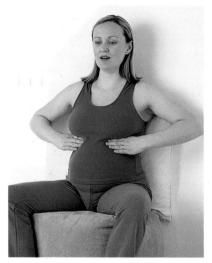

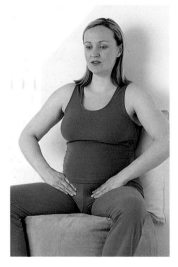

1 Sit in a comfortable position with your back supported, your knees apart and your feet flat on the floor. Place your hands on your upper chest with your elbows out at either side. Breathing naturally, pull your elbows down to lift and expand your chest as you exhale.

2 Lower your hands and place them on your rib cage. Keep your elbows out, push your ribs out under your hands as you inhale, and then press your hands gently inwards as you exhale. Feel that you are breathing out in a straight line up your spine. Relax any tense areas in your back.

3 Place your hands on the tops of your thighs so that your hands adjoin your pubic bone. Exhale to the base of your spine to utilize your lower abdominal muscles and pelvic floor muscles in the flow of your breath.

MUDRAS

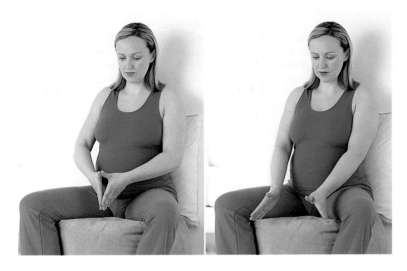

Gentle opener Sit up straight with your back well supported. Position your hands in front of you, fingers pointing down, and make a triangle by joining your thumbs, your fingertips and the base of your index fingers. Exhale and move your hands downwards and out. This bold, opening hand gesture is symbolic of your birth canal opening wide.

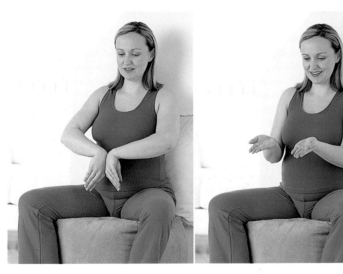

Receiving & giving Position your hands out flat in front of you with your thumbs tucked under. Turn your wrists in so that the backs of your hands touch. Rotate them down and back up several times. End with an open gesture.

Unconditional love Relax and breathe evenly, holding your hands against your chest in Prayer pose. Without moving your elbows, exhale and gently open your forearms out with your palms facing up in a gesture of unconditional love. All mudras can either be held while you breathe freely, or repeated slowly or rapidly several times.

BREATHING TECHNIQUES

These exercises are best practised after you have completed your Section breathing *(p82)*. Like Section breathing, they involve the flow of breath and energy as you contract and release your muscles, particularly in the lower part of the abdomen and the back. Such simple techniques deepen your breathing and help you to gain confidence in your ability to give birth lightly using effective breathing. You can also use these exercises to wind down after your yoga routine and before relaxation.

> **CAUTIONS** For breathing exercises in a seated position:
> • Use a chair or sit against a wall with a cushion to support your lower back if you cannot sit comfortably on the floor.
> • Do not use your pelvic floor muscles in these exercises; actively relax your pelvic floor during each exhalation in preparation for birth.

BASIC BREATHING

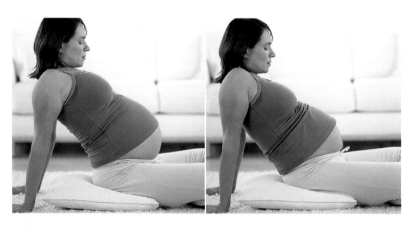

Sit on a cushion on the floor with your feet in Butterfly pose. Place your hands on the floor behind you. Breathe in, open out your chest and draw your shoulder blades together. Then gently tilt your pelvis back and press down on your sitting bones as you exhale slowly.

STRONG & SPACIOUS

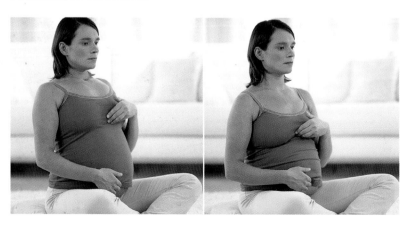

Sit upright on a cushion. Place one hand at your sternum and the other by your pubic bone. Inhale and push your sternum up slowly while applying a gentle pressure on your pubic bone with your hand. Sustain this double action as you exhale. Repeat three times. Stop if you feel light-headed.

POWER PELVIC BREATHING

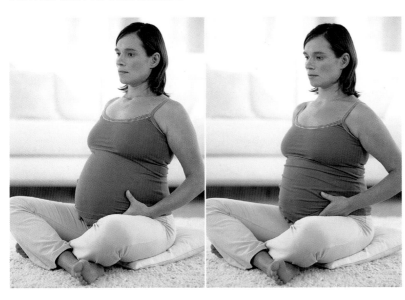

Sit upright on a cushion, legs crossed, with your hands on your lower abdomen. Inhale deeply. Draw your exhalation out by pushing down into your lower abdomen. Register the pressure that builds at the base of your spine. Aim to release this pressure and relax all the muscles of your pelvic floor as you complete your exhalation. Let your lungs fill out again effortlessly before your next "power breath". Repeat three times.

STANDING PELVIC BREATHING

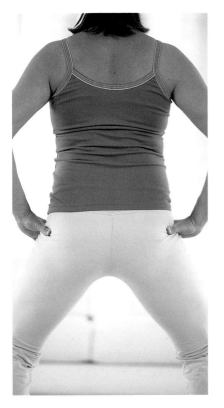

Stand in Mountain pose with your feet apart and your knees slightly bent. As you inhale, contract your buttock muscles as tightly as you can. Exhale, release your buttock muscles and bend your knees, keeping your spine straight. This action is essential in making way for your baby during birth. Notice the synchronized toning of your lower abdominal muscles.

BLOWING A FEATHER

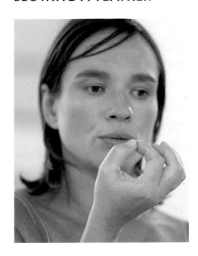

Bring one hand to your mouth and join your thumb and index finger. Without contracting your abdominal muscles, purse your lips, inhale, and as you exhale, emit a voiceless "Hoo" sound. Feel your out-breath cooling your fingers. This may be helpful during labour.

ACTIVE RELAXATION
Viparita Karani

Every yoga pose offers a balance of activity and relaxation, of doing and being, so relaxation exercises are essential for the completion of a yoga routine, however short it may be. If you are new to yoga and still feel unsure about your ability to relax deeply, use these stretches and the rhythm of your breathing to lead you into relaxation. These skills will be a great resource in late pregnancy and after your baby is born to rapidly recharge and refresh yourself.

BENEFITS AND CAUTIONS
Relaxation poses induce a deep rest that has positive effects on the endocrine and nervous systems.

Do not practise this sequence after thirty weeks unless you raise your lower back from the floor to avoid pressure on the vena cava.

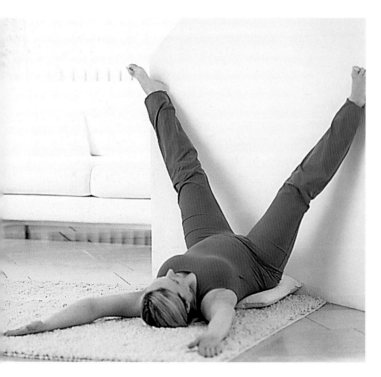

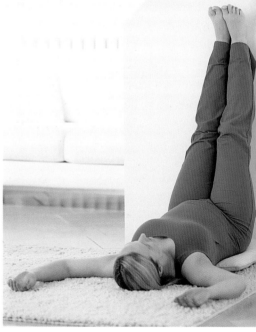

1 Sit on a cushion parallel to a wall. Swivel round on your bottom until your legs and bottom are against the wall and your back is flat on the floor. Open your legs out comfortably so that your inner thighs are relaxed, and extend your arms along the floor behind your head. Stretch in this position for six deep breaths.

2 On the last out-breath, bring your legs together and relax your arms. Continue to breathe deeply as you focus your awareness on your chest and upper back, and abdomen and lower back, for six breaths. Release tension in your shoulders and back as you exhale.

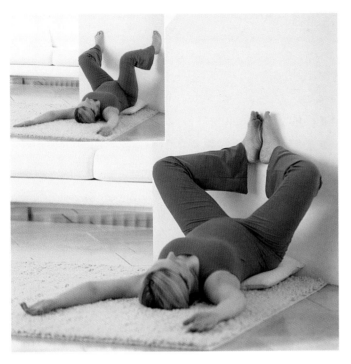

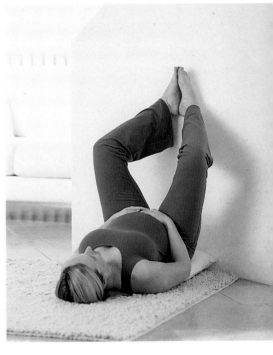

3 Bend your knees and place your feet flat against the wall. As you exhale, push your heels against the wall slightly while pressing the base of your spine down to relax the deeper pelvic muscles. Practise three times. Then rest with your feet in Butterfly pose and your knees open comfortably to each side. Hold for six breaths, releasing any tightness in the pelvis and groin with each out-breath.

4 Keeping your joined feet against the wall, find a position that is most relaxing for your legs, or place your feet on a bean bag or a pouffe. Place your hands around your abdomen to create a circle of energy that you and your baby can enjoy. Hold for six breaths.

5 Always roll onto one side with your knees bent to come out of this pose. Kneel up on all fours and stretch your back for a few seconds before standing up slowly.

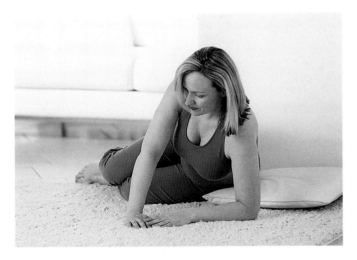

WORK IN THE POSE

Experience the difference between stretching your arms out to expand and strengthen your breathing capacity, and placing your hands softly on your abdomen to relax your arms and body in a restful pose.

RELAXATION

Relaxation is an integral part of yoga. A full relaxation of 20 minutes or more brings special benefits, which are particularly desirable in pregnancy. Going deep inside yourself allows you to access inner peace and intuition beyond the daily hustle and bustle and the roller coaster of normal, yet often trying, emotions that occur during any pregnancy. Nurturing yourself through relaxation will allow you to store precious reserves of energy and respond better to the demands of your new baby. It will also help you to be calmly assertive and receive any offers of help gracefully.

ADAPTED CORPSE POSE Shavasana

1 Find a quiet environment where you will not be disturbed. Use cushions and a blanket to make yourself warm and comfortable. Lie on the floor or on a firm bed and bend your knees to align your spine. *Between 28–32 weeks use a cushion to raise your lower back, but after 32 weeks of pregnancy avoid relaxing in any supine position.*

2 Relax your lower jaw and ensure that the base of your neck is aligned. Use a cushion under your neck for support if needed so that you can look up vertically without strain. Close your eyes and breathe deeply for three breaths, using each exhalation to let go of any tension.

3 Passively register any thoughts or emotions, as if projected on a white screen, that enter your mind. Trust that negative emotions are not part of you, just projections on the screen. Relax the palms of your hands to open and soften your heart.

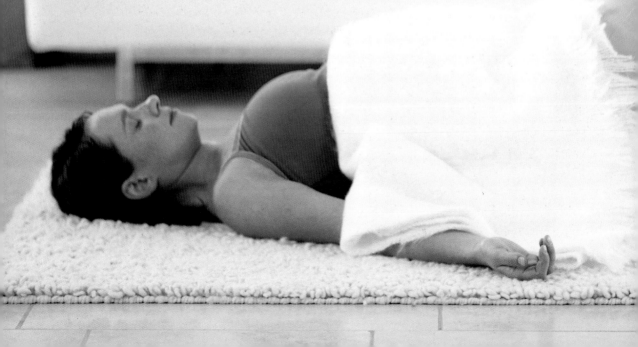

ROLLING UP

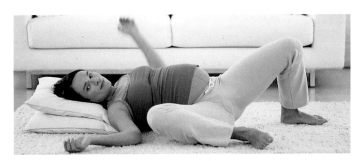

1 From lying on your back with your knees bent, roll to the right and bring your right knee up to waist level. Bend your right elbow and position it on the floor by your right knee.

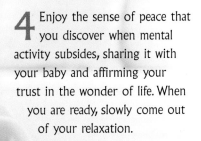

4 Enjoy the sense of peace that you discover when mental activity subsides, sharing it with your baby and affirming your trust in the wonder of life. When you are ready, slowly come out of your relaxation.

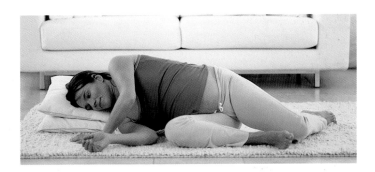

2 Place the palm of your left hand on the floor at shoulder level and ensure that it is aligned with your bent knee. Keep your neck soft as you roll onto your right side.

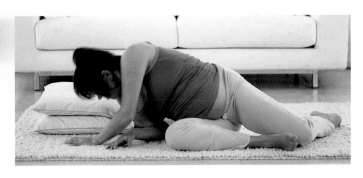

3 Shift your weight onto your left hand and knee. Then bring your right knee underneath your right hip, and your right hand underneath your right shoulder. Come up into an all-fours position, from which you can stand up slowly without strain.

SPECIAL APPLICATIONS

Many of the common discomforts of pregnancy can be alleviated by applying movements that relieve pressure on aching parts of the body, and then strengthen the surrounding muscles. Yoga is most effective in its ability to tone the inner skeletal muscles, which we are not normally aware of when we practise other forms of exercise. The use of deep breathing in these special applications will help you not only relieve the pain, but gain long-term awareness and control of the pelvic muscles, which are important to your well-being at all ages of your adult life.

SYMPHYSIS PUBIS DISORDER (SPD)

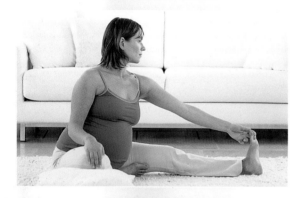

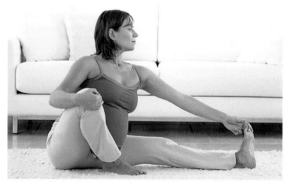

1 Sit tall on the floor with your legs extended. Bend your right knee and rest it on the floor or on a cushion for support. Place your right heel by your groin. Hold your left big toe with your left hand (use a belt if necessary). Breathe deeply for six breaths.

2 Keep hold of your left toe with your left hand and raise your right knee. Position your foot on the floor, as close to your body as you can, and hold your knee with your right hand. Breathe deeply for six breaths. Repeat both stretches on the other side.

CARPAL TUNNEL SYNDROME

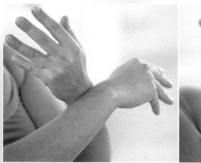

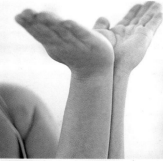

Sit or stand. Cross your wrists so that they touch and circle your hands forwards, then backwards, six times. Wiggle your fingers throughout. Breathe evenly. Then join your elbows, lower arms and the heels of your hands. Inhale and stretch your fingers as you open your hands. Exhale and close your hands. Repeat three times.

BACKACHE

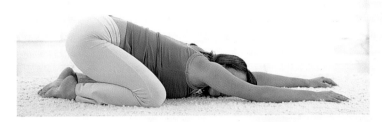

1 Position yourself in extended Child's pose on the floor: knees bent and opened out, arms extended, palms pressing down, and with your head resting to one side. Then come onto all fours.

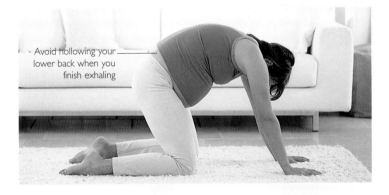

Avoid hollowing your lower back when you finish exhaling

2 Inhale, lift your shoulders high and relax your head down in Cat pose. Exhale, stretch between your shoulder blades and lengthen the base of your spine towards your heels. Repeat slowly three times.

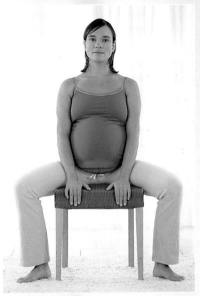

Weak lower back Sit tall on a chair with your knees wide apart. Place your hands at the front of the chair, take a breath and push down with your hands as you exhale. Keep your perineum relaxed. Feel a build-up of energy and heat in your back and abdomen as you breathe for six cycles.

SUPPORTED RELAXATION

Arrange two cushions on the floor next to a pouffe or bean bag, then lie on your back so that the cushions support your lumbar spine and hips and the pouffe supports your legs. Position your feet in Butterfly pose, rest your hands on your lower abdomen, close your eyes and relax, breathing deeply.

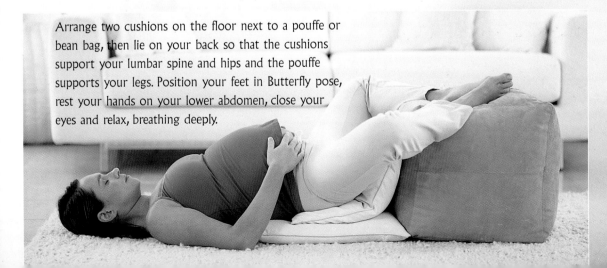

WEAK BLADDER

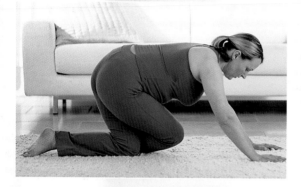
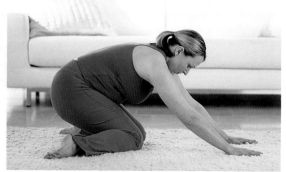

1 Position yourself on all fours. Use a cushion if you need to support your knees. Cross your right leg over your left leg and redistribute your weight equally between your hands and left knee. Breathe deeply for six breaths, drawing your pelvic floor muscles up as you inhale, then even further up as you exhale.

2 Return to an all-fours position. Bring your knees together while keeping your feet apart. Move your weight back towards your heels, using a cushion to sit on if you wish. Breathe deeply for six breaths, lifting your pelvic floor muscles in the same way as step 1. Repeat steps 1 and 2 three times a day.

HAEMORRHOIDS

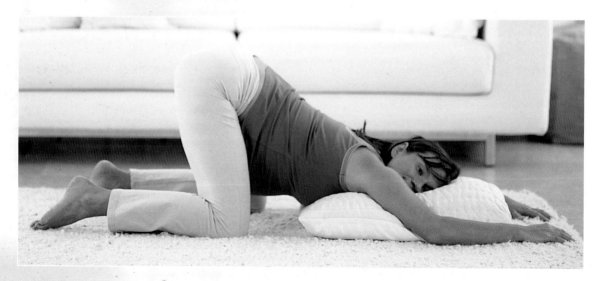

Position yourself on all fours. Place a large cushion in front of you, lean forwards from your hips, turn your head to one side and rest it on the cushion. Let your arms rest on the floor. Make sure that your head and shoulders are also relaxed. As you inhale, tighten your anal sphincter as much as you can. Exhale and release slowly. Repeat 12 times. Do not be discouraged if you feel very little movement at first as you breathe in and out. Practise daily, morning and evening. Continue even if you feel there is a definite improvement.

SCIATICA

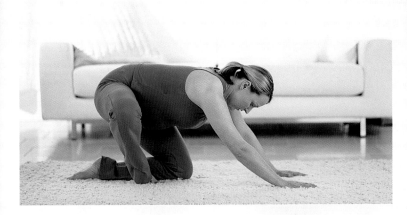

1 Begin on all fours. Place a cushion under your left foot for comfort if needed. Move your hips back and rest your weight on your left leg. Bring your right foot forwards so that you balance on the front of your foot. Swing your hips gently from left to right, or make small circles with your right knee. Practise more circles on the affected side. Avoid this first step if the pain is acute.

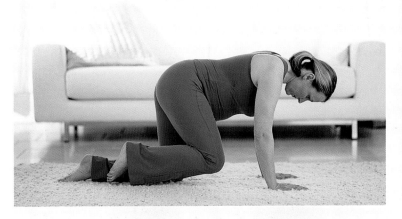

2 Practise this step to prevent and relieve the pain. Start in a steady all-fours position. Move your weight towards your hands. Slowly raise your right leg off the floor slightly, keeping your knee bent and your hips level. Bring your right knee forwards and make small circles at floor level with your knee. Keep your foot relaxed and breathe evenly.

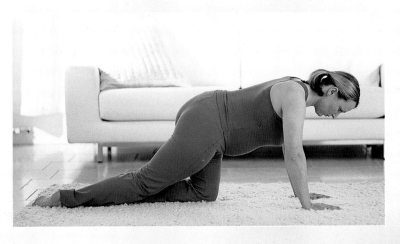

3 This action relieves acute pain. Let your right leg sink to the floor and relax it completely as you drop your right hip. Shake your right leg loosely from your hip to your toes. Breathe deeply through this movement for two or three minutes, expanding your exhalation to release pressure on the sciatic nerve. Voice your exhalation with a deep "Aaah" sound if this helps.

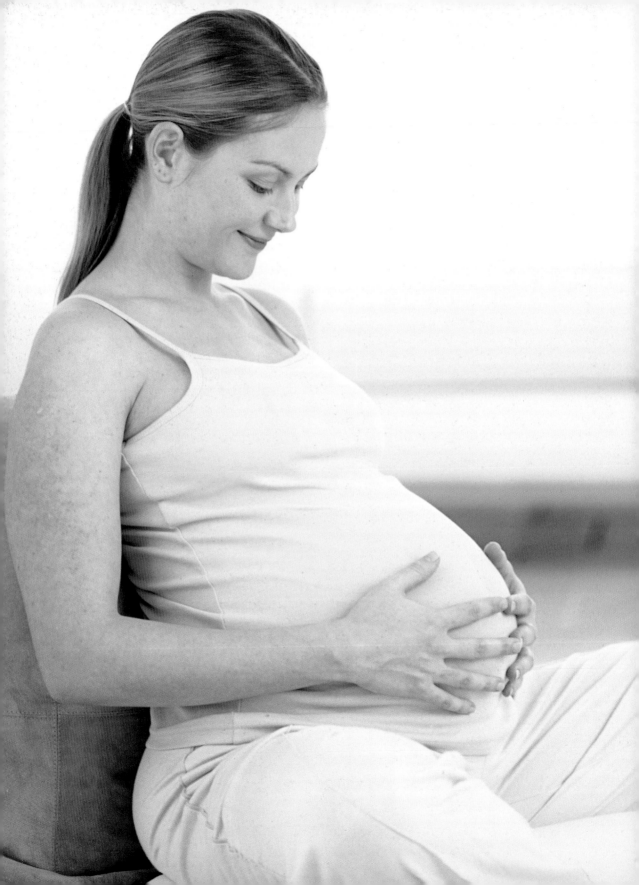

LATE
PREGNANCY
34 TO 40+ WEEKS

During the last weeks of pregnancy your baby actively prepares to be born, so getting ready for this arrival becomes your main focus. Your priorities are to keep yourself fit, comfortable and relaxed. Yoga postures and breathing will prepare you physically, mentally and spiritually for labour, greatly empowering you from within. However your birth may unfold, yoga will help you stay centred and connected with your baby.

"Full and free, vibrant with energy, how extraordinary the joy that wells up from the depth of my Self!"
Frederick Leboyer, *Birth without Violence*

ALIGNMENT OF SPINE

Now that you are carrying a heavier baby, your posture is more important than ever. Aligning your spine daily with simple stretches will instantly energize and refresh you, and also benefit your baby. Be aware that although lying back on soft furniture may seem relaxing, it actually slows down the circulation of blood to the placenta and could encourage your baby to move into a position that is less advantageous for birth.

> **CAUTIONS** Adapt the pose if:
> • You have varicose veins. Practise all these poses in a sitting position.
> • You have high blood pressure. Don't attempt to raise your arms above your head, even though deep breathing with horizontal arm stretches can sometimes help to reduce this condition.

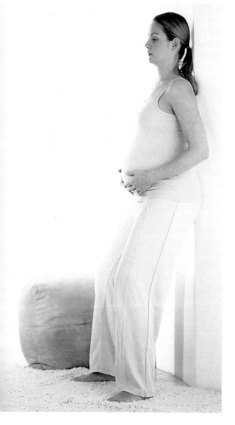 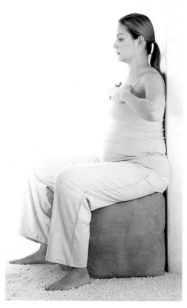 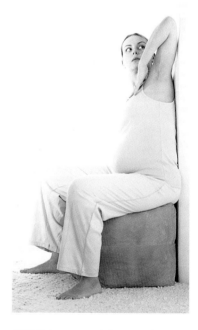

1 Stand a short distance from a wall. Bend your knees slightly and rest the length of your back against the wall. Breathe deeply.

2 Sit tall on a pouffe or stool positioned against a wall. Move your knees and feet hip-width apart and align your back fully. Then place your hands on your clavicles (collarbone) and open your upper chest to create more breathing space.

3 Relax your right arm down and lift your left elbow up against the wall by the side of your head. Keep your left hand on your clavicle. Gently turn your head to look at your elbow and breathe deeply for four breaths. Repeat on the right side.

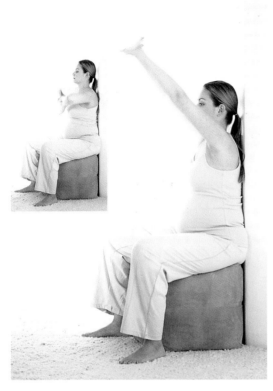

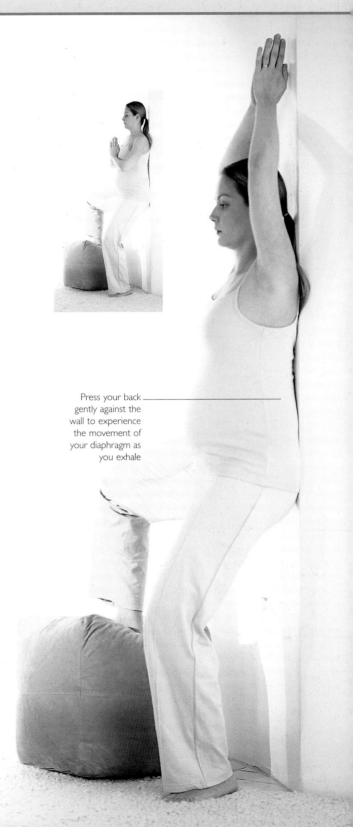

Press your back gently against the wall to experience the movement of your diaphragm as you exhale

4 Interlock your fingers at chest height. Turn your hands out, inhale and extend your arms out as you exhale. Raise your arms only as high as feels comfortable while keeping your back aligned against the wall. Breathe deeply for four breaths. Then bend your elbows, lower your arms down slowly and release your fingers.

5 Stand up, bend your left knee slightly and place your right foot on the pouffe. Align your back against the wall and join your hands in Prayer pose at chest height. Breathe deeply. As you inhale, raise your hands up slowly. Exhale, keeping your elbows bent, and extend your arms fully only if your back remains aligned against the wall. Then lower your hands and relax.

SUN SALUTATION
Surya Namaskar

In this adapted Sun salutation for late pregnancy, your priorities are to protect your lower back and to build strength in your pelvic and leg muscles so that they can easily carry the extra weight of your baby. Continue to enjoy moving around right up to labour as you create more space inside for your baby: stretch up to the sky and ground yourself in time to the rhythm of your breathing.

> **CAUTIONS** Practise this Sun salutation sequence slowly:
> • Don't hold any position too long; keep your movements flowing.
> • If bending forwards makes you feel light-headed, or if raised blood pressure is a concern, skip steps 4–7.

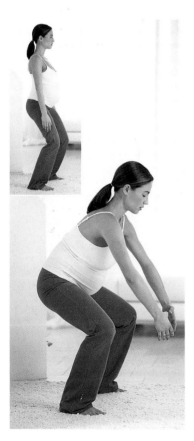

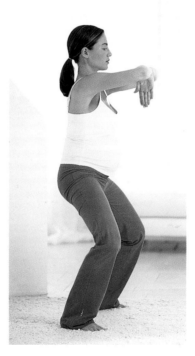

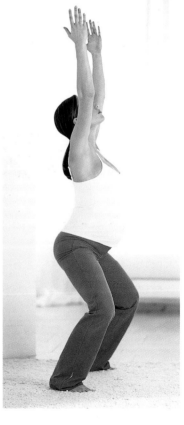

1 Stand wide in Mountain pose with your knees bent. Exhale and lower yourself into a semi-squat, as if gathering up flowers.

2 Raise your imaginary bunch of flowers slowly to chest level as you inhale up. Then turn your hands so that they are positioned back to back as you exhale. Keep your knees bent and stand strong with a straight back.

3 Take a deep breath and lift your arms up as if you were throwing your flowers into the sky. Exhale in the stretch.

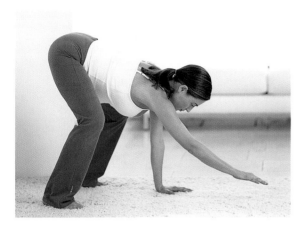

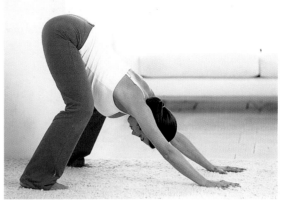

4 Inhale, then on your out-breath lower yourself into a semi-squat. Place one hand on the floor and walk your hands forwards along the floor in front of you, keeping them shoulder-width apart.

5 Keep your knees bent and your heels on the floor as you stretch through your spine and arms in this wide Dog pose. Hold the stretch for a full cycle of breathing.

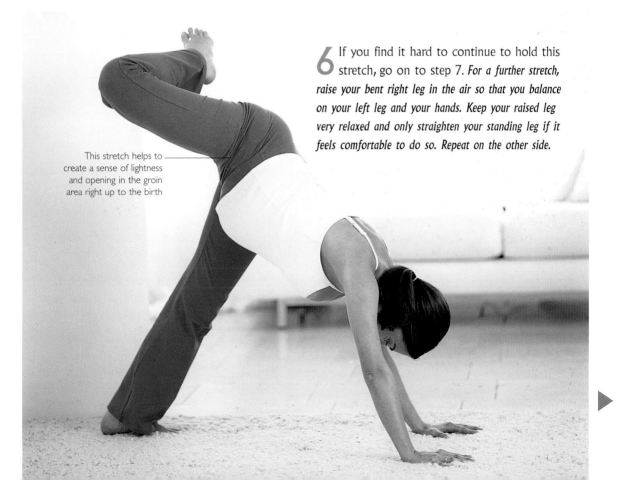

This stretch helps to create a sense of lightness and opening in the groin area right up to the birth

6 If you find it hard to continue to hold this stretch, go on to step 7. *For a further stretch, raise your bent right leg in the air so that you balance on your left leg and your hands. Keep your raised leg very relaxed and only straighten your standing leg if it feels comfortable to do so. Repeat on the other side.*

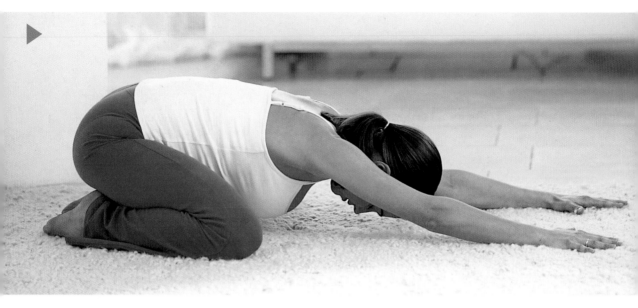

7 Lower your raised leg, then go down onto all fours. Rest in Child's pose with your knees positioned wide apart to make space for your baby. Release the base of your spine downwards towards your heels to elongate your back, and hold the pose for two breaths. Exhale fully before moving back onto all fours on your next inhalation. *If keeping your arms fully extended on the floor causes some tension in your shoulders, lean forwards to rest on your elbows and forearms instead.*

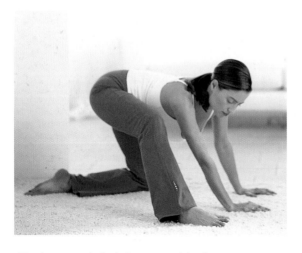

8 As you exhale, bring your right foot out to the side, placing it on the floor wherever it feels comfortable. Rotate your knee outwards with a flowing movement of your whole torso as you breathe in and out. Repeat on the left side.

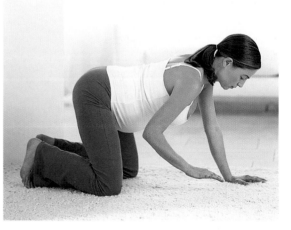

9 Return to a steady all-fours position and check that your hands and knees are correctly aligned. Turn your toes under and slowly walk your hands back to your knees until your weight tips your body towards your heels and into a squat position.

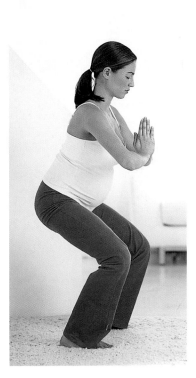

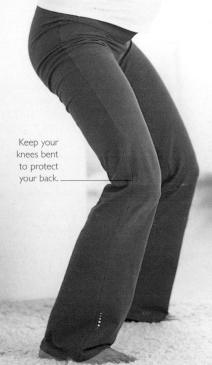

Open your
shoulders as
much as you
can by rotating
your armpits
outwards

Keep your
knees bent
to protect
your back.

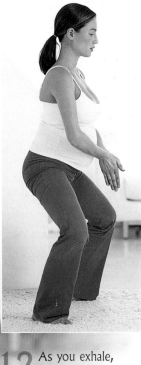

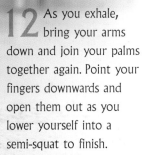

10 Use the momentum of
your squatting movement
to stand up on an in-breath. Keep
your knees bent and join your
hands in Prayer pose as you
exhale. Make sure that you keep
the base of your palms joined.

11 On your next in-breath,
extend your arms upwards,
opening your chest fully as you
separate your hands and stretch
into your fingertips. *If stretching
your arms causes tension, keep your
elbows slightly bent.*

12 As you exhale,
bring your arms
down and join your palms
together again. Point your
fingers downwards and
open them out as you
lower yourself into a
semi-squat to finish.

CIRCULAR STRETCHES

By late pregnancy, your centre of gravity lies deep within your pelvis. Circular stretches, with their harmonious rhythms around your baby's body, will help to open up your hips and pelvic area. Performing these spinal movements while remaining steady in a wide standing position will also increase your stamina and poise. Provided you keep your knees bent, these rotations can even become an energetic dance that will help to revitalize you.

BENEFITS Express your vitality with movements that suit your very pregnant body:
• Circular movements help to increase your awareness of the pull of gravity.
• In spite of your heaviness, these poses are fun and show you how to exercise with grace and energy.

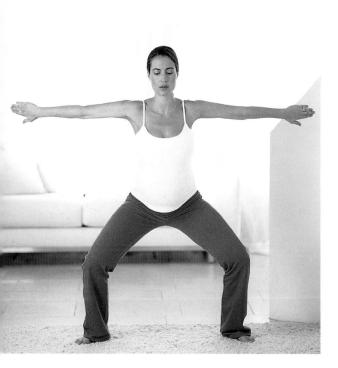

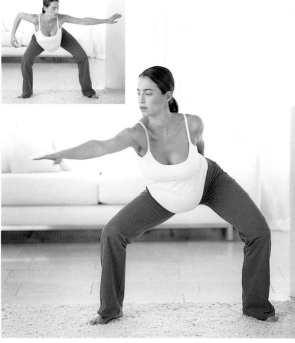

1 Stand wide in Mountain pose and bend your knees, keeping your back straight. Turn your feet out 45°. Inhale and extend your arms straight out in front of your chest, palms facing down. As you exhale, stretch your arms out to each side with your palms facing backwards.

2 Inhale and stretch your right arm out above your right knee. As you exhale, make a wide semi-circle with your hand and reach out behind without moving your hips. Follow your hand with a wide twist of your shoulders. Bend your right arm in at the end of the movement, then stretch your left arm forwards on the next in-breath to repeat the semi-circle.

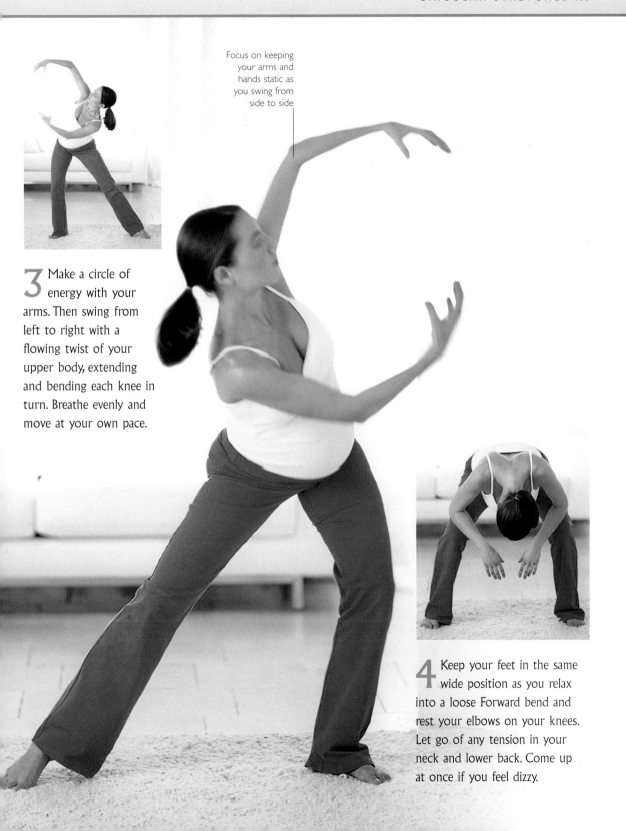

Focus on keeping your arms and hands static as you swing from side to side

3 Make a circle of energy with your arms. Then swing from left to right with a flowing twist of your upper body, extending and bending each knee in turn. Breathe evenly and move at your own pace.

4 Keep your feet in the same wide position as you relax into a loose Forward bend and rest your elbows on your knees. Let go of any tension in your neck and lower back. Come up at once if you feel dizzy.

WARRIOR TO WALL
Adapted Virabhadrasana

Warrior poses generate immense energy. Directing this energy in late pregnancy to control and release the pelvic muscles is helpful preparation for labour. As well as literally offering your body a strong support, the Wall can help you to draw inner strength right up to labour. Whether you are experienced or new to yoga, these stretches increase your awareness of the power of your breathing.

BENEFITS These poses help to:
- Strengthen your back muscles.
- Involve the muscles of the back and abdomen in deep breathing.
- Stretch hamstring and calf muscles.
- Lift the inner arches of your feet to relieve pressure on the pelvis.

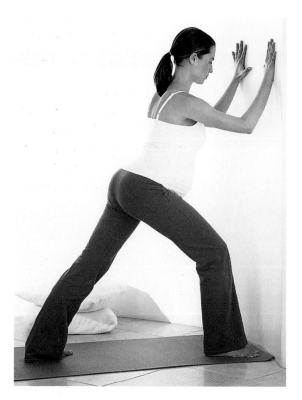

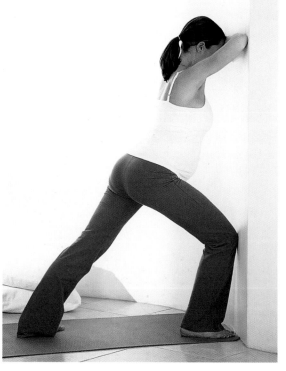

1 Stand facing a wall so that your forearms can rest comfortably against the wall. Take your left leg back and bend your right knee forwards, keeping your hips aligned. Take four breaths, pressing your hands against the wall on each out-breath.

2 Cross your forearms and rest your elbows against the wall so that your arms can support your forehead. Keep your left foot in place and lean your right knee against the wall. Enjoy the expansion of your rib cage as you take four deep breaths.

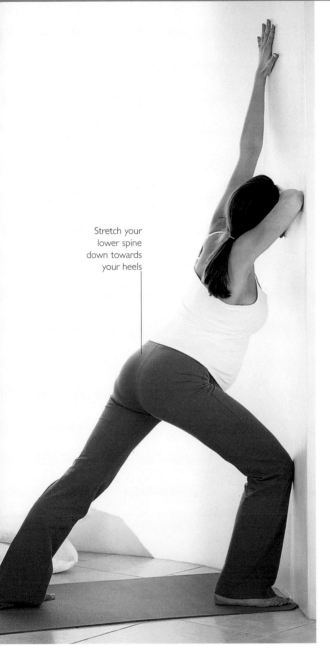

Stretch your
lower spine
down towards
your heels

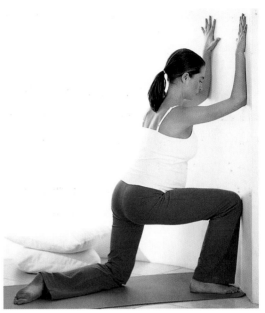

4 Keep your right leg in position and kneel down on your left knee. Place a cushion under your knee for comfort if needed. Lower your hands so that your forearms rest vertically against the wall. Tuck your tail bone in to relax your lower back, and breathe deeply for four breaths.

Use cushions under
your feet and your
head to help you relax

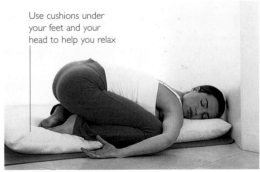

3 On an in-breath, extend your left arm vertically up the wall by your left ear while keeping your right elbow in place. Exhale and stretch further into your fingertips as you press your left heel onto the floor and focus on keeping your right side totally relaxed.

5 After this vigorous breathing, rest on cushions in Turtle pose with your knees open wide, arms folded around your knees and your head to one side. *If you do not enjoy Turtle pose, try Child's pose.* Then repeat the sequence on the other side.

YOGA DANCES

Adapted Indian dance movements and the dynamic stillness of held poses – similar to those displayed by Indian gods and goddesses in statues and pictures – can help to make you supple, light-hearted and full of joyous energy with which to welcome your baby. As you make all the necessary preparations for the birth, use these fluid movements, performed in strong standing positions, to simply enjoy your creativity at this special time.

SHAKTI DANCE

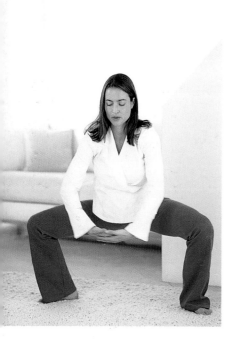

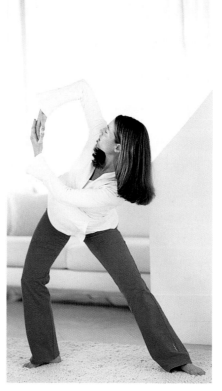

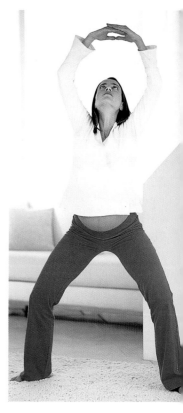

1 Stand with feet wide apart. Place one hand over the other. Lower into a semi-squat. Press your hands down rhythmically in small circles, moving your shoulders freely.

2 Keep your feet and hands in position as you draw your elbows from side to side to make wide semi-circles. Bend your knees to drop down in the middle of each swinging motion.

3 If you feel confident, complete a full circle by raising your elbows up over your head and then down on the other side.

SNAKE DANCE

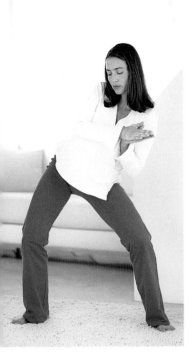

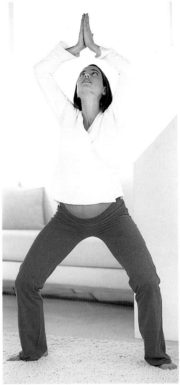

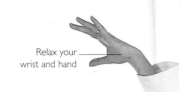

Relax your wrist and hand

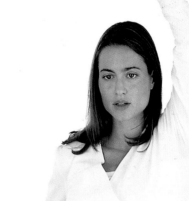

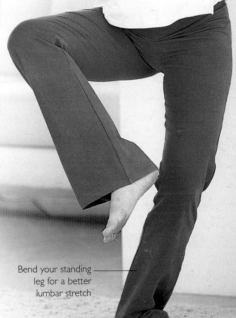

Bend your standing leg for a better lumbar stretch

1 Maintain a strong standing base with your knees bent. Join your palms and move your shoulders and elbows rhythmically as you point your fingers left, then right. Moving in a figure of eight also helps to mobilize your lower back.

2 Once you feel confident with your hand movements, move your "snake" hands up and down in front of your body in a flowing dance. Look up at your hands as you raise your arms above your head, and keep your knees bent as you reach downwards.

SHIVA DANCE

Stand tall and open your right knee out to the side. Rest your right heel on your left leg wherever it feels most comfortable. At the same time, bring your left arm up above your head and keep your right arm relaxed. Breathe evenly. Swap your legs and arms in a rhythm that suits you.

SITTING STRETCHES

Sitting on a firm but comfortable seat to stretch in late pregnancy ensures that there is no compression in your lower back and abdomen. While you are grounded in this position, your stretches can extend through the whole spine and your breathing can travel easily down to your perineum. Thus, what was initially a relaxed stretch for gaining awareness of the perineum in early pregnancy *(pp.32–33)* now becomes a powerfully effective breathing technique with gentle movements that will make the best possible use of gravity when bearing down at the birth.

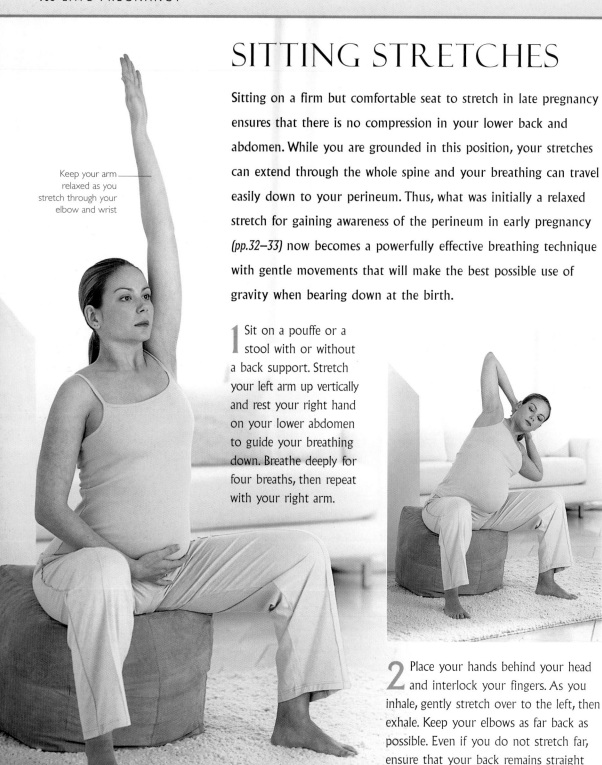

Keep your arm relaxed as you stretch through your elbow and wrist

1 Sit on a pouffe or a stool with or without a back support. Stretch your left arm up vertically and rest your right hand on your lower abdomen to guide your breathing down. Breathe deeply for four breaths, then repeat with your right arm.

2 Place your hands behind your head and interlock your fingers. As you inhale, gently stretch over to the left, then exhale. Keep your elbows as far back as possible. Even if you do not stretch far, ensure that your back remains straight at all times. Repeat twice on each side.

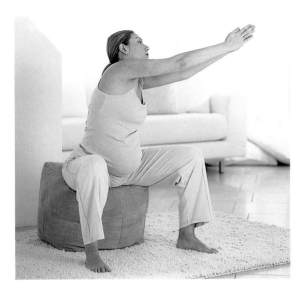

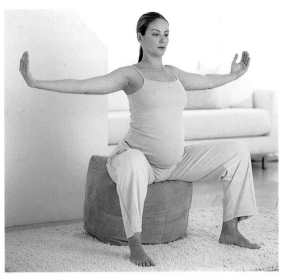

3 Extend your arms out in front of you and join the palms of your hands. As you exhale, stretch your arms over to the left, then on your next out-breath stretch over to the right. Repeat twice.

4 Open your extended arms out to the sides of your body as you inhale, then turn the backs of your hands out in a wide receiving gesture as you exhale. Make sure that you don't arch your back.

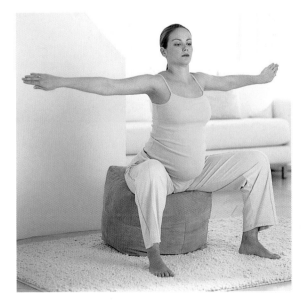

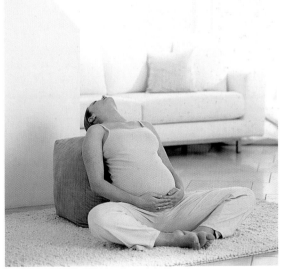

5 On your next out-breath, turn your hands so that your palms face backwards. Breathe evenly, turning your wrists forwards and back, and feel the muscles of your back and abdomen working.

6 Use a soft but firm support to relax in Butterfly pose (p.21) and breathe deeply. If this feels comfortable, release your neck back and rest in a supported neck stretch to complete the sequence.

WIDE KNEELING STRETCHES

Kneeling is one of the best positions you can adopt at this stage of your pregnancy. In this position you can stretch your spine properly with your coccyx free from pressure, since the weight of your uterus is taken by your legs, elbows and hands making contact with the floor. Your baby can also benefit from the maximum amount of space in your pelvis when your knees are wide apart. Practise these poses too if you wish to prepare for a birthing position on all fours.

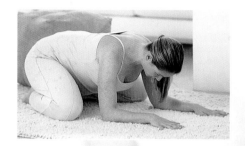

1 Position yourself in a wide Cat pose on the floor: move your knees apart, bend your arms and rest your forearms flat on the floor in line with your knees.

2 Raise your buttocks and, with your weight evenly balanced and your spine and head aligned, inhale and extend your right arm up vertically. Press your left elbow and your right knee onto the floor. Turn the palm of your hand out as you exhale.

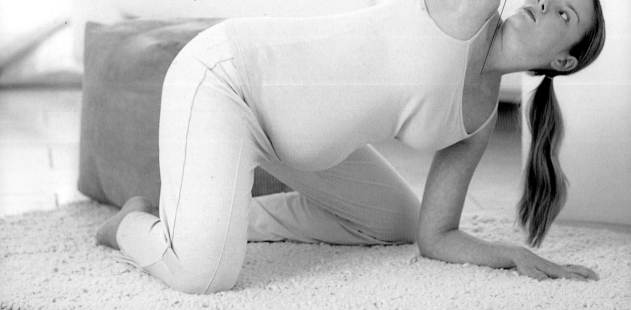

Keep your arm relaxed and point your fingers

Try to stretch up from under your shoulder blades and sternum

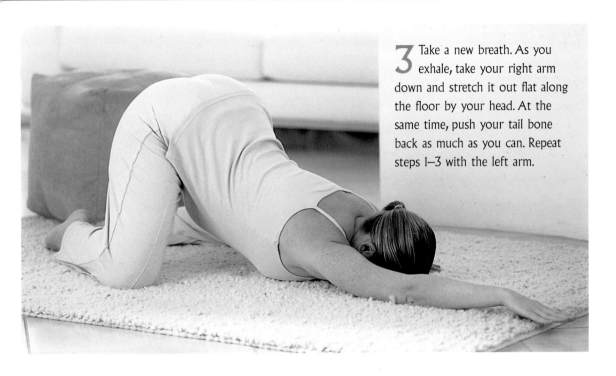

3 Take a new breath. As you exhale, take your right arm down and stretch it out flat along the floor by your head. At the same time, push your tail bone back as much as you can. Repeat steps 1–3 with the left arm.

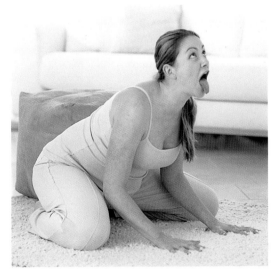

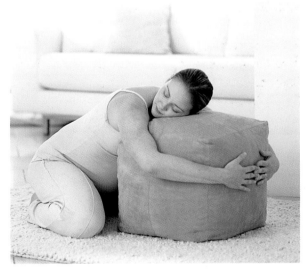

4 Sit back on your heels and rest your hands on the floor in front of your knees. Inhale and put your tongue out fiercely as you exhale in Lion pose, perhaps accompanied by a deep roaring sound. Use this pose to rid yourself of any inevitable irrational fears before labour.

5 Resting in a supported kneeling position at an angle of 30–45° is ideal to ensure that your baby has the widest space in which to enter the birth canal. Keep your knees wide apart and relax your upper body, arms and head against your support. Use cushions under your feet and knees if needed in this popular labour position.

YOGA FOR BETTER SLEEP

Lighter, interrupted sleep affects most women in late pregnancy. This is usually due to hormonal changes and the increased weight of your baby, so gentle, loosening movements are needed to help release the lumbar and cervical areas of the spine. Making simple adjustments to your sleeping positions can also be very effective in promoting better sleep and deep rest before labour.

WOBBLE & RELAX

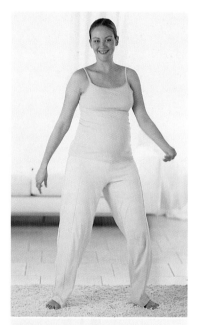

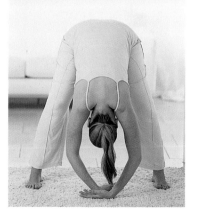

CAMEL WALK

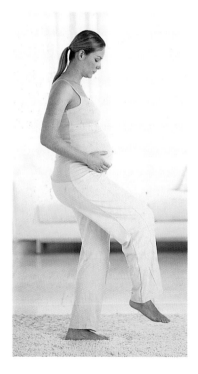

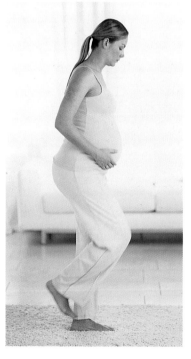

1 Stand with your knees bent and tip your pelvis forwards. Hold your abdomen and continue to rotate your pelvis from front to back, shifting your weight from one leg to the other, as you walk in a straight line.

2 Whether you walk forwards or backwards using this camel-like step, try to turn your movements into an easy, smooth, flowing wave that extends up to your shoulders and neck. Breathe evenly throughout.

Stand with your arms loose and relaxed. Zigzag your shoulders and hips down in a hilarious wobble effect as you bend your knees, and then come up again. Finish in a Forward bend, hanging from your hips like a rag doll.

SLEEPING POSITIONS

1 Lie on the bed on your left side. Bend your left knee and bring it up to hip level to rest on two pillows. Make sure that your spine is comfortably aligned, and avoid high pillows. Lying on your left side may further encourage your baby to adopt an optimal presentation for birth.

Adjust the angle of your leg to elongate your spine

BENEFITS Your baby may now press uncomfortably on nerves and blood vessels. Relieve discomfort by:
• Sleeping mainly on your side.
• Strategically placing cushions to avoid compression, keep your spine aligned and aid comfortable sleep.

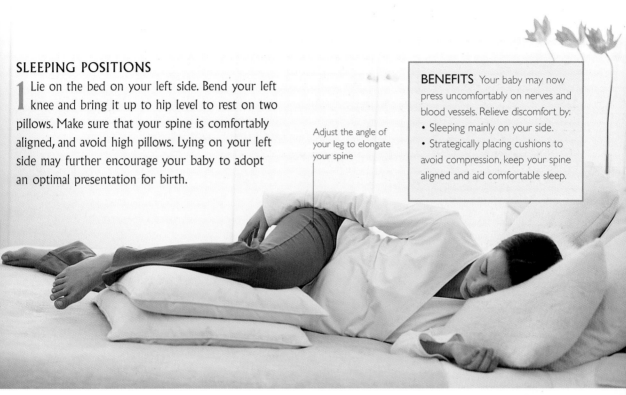

2 If you want to sleep on your back without discomfort or possible risks to your baby, extend one leg and place a small cushion under your hip so that your body is tilted in a three-quarter supine position. Bend your other leg and place a pillow under your knee. Use your early pregnancy spinal rolls (p.23) to move comfortably from one side to the other with minimal disturbance to your sleep.

Place a small cushion under your sacrum to the side of your extended leg

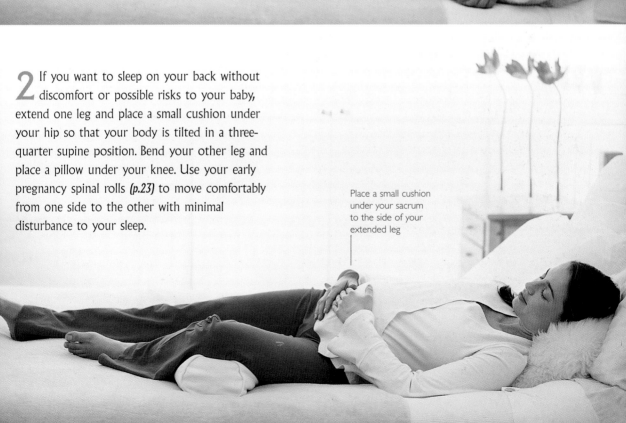

STRETCHING FOR BIRTH

Labour pains are often exacerbated by either lower backache or lower abdominal cramps. These stretching sequences aim to create greater mobility around the tail bone and groin area by means of deep breathing using the pelvic floor muscles and the skeletal muscles. This action can also help your baby's head to engage. Modifying these stretches to suit your individual level of fitness will still produce excellent results.

CAUTIONS Leave out any birthing stretches that you do not feel completely comfortable with. If you have been affected by SPD at any time during your pregnancy, do not practise deep squats. Instead, sit down slowly on a low chair or stool, keeping your back straight at all times.

LOW ROCKING SEQUENCE

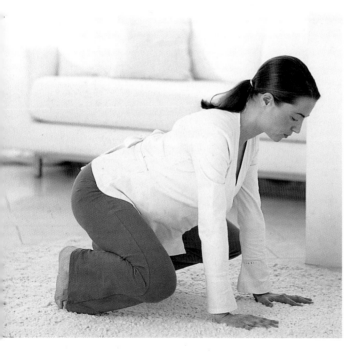

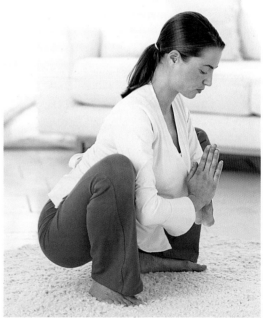

1 Start in a kneeling position, sitting on your heels with your hands on the floor in front of your knees. Breathe deeply to ease any discomfort in your lower back. Come onto your toes and lift one knee slightly. Make small rocking movements with your pelvis, back and forth and sideways, to create more space around your tail bone.

2 Amplify this rocking motion with a greater movement, to the point where you can move into a deep squatting position if you wish. Squat only if you find it easy to hold this position with your heels on the floor and your back straight. Breathe deeply. *Alternatively, rock forwards again.*

WIDE PELVIC STRETCH & TWIST

1 Sit on the floor or a cushion, extend your left leg and turn your toes up. Bend your right leg and place your right foot on the floor. Lean forwards and hook two fingers around your left big toe, or use a yoga belt. Lift your pelvic floor muscles as you inhale, and relax them on a long out-breath.

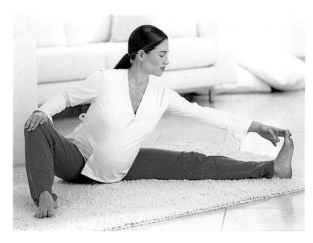

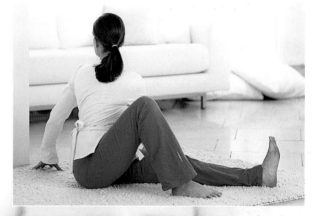

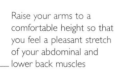
Raise your arms to a comfortable height so that you feel a pleasant stretch of your abdominal and lower back muscles

2 Bring your bent right leg round so that it is parallel with your extended left leg. Turn to your left and place your hands on the floor wherever it feels comfortable. Breathing deeply in this gentle twist irrigates your lower abdomen with fresh blood and massages your baby.

3 If you feel confident, roll round to your right side and, keeping your right leg bent, bring it in close to your body. Breathe deeply, relaxing your pelvic muscles, then exhale in an upward arm stretch. Repeat steps 1–3 on the other side.

BIRTHING VISUALIZATION
Dhyana

Throughout pregnancy, your breathing has connected you with your baby. Having used yoga breathing to increase your awareness, you can now make full use of helpful techniques to experience a "light" birth. Explore the power and benefits of breathing, sound and visualization together before you begin birthing contractions.

> **BENEFITS** Breathing helps to:
> • Conserve energy, create rhythm during labour and get rid of tension as contractions come and go.
> • Breathe your baby out into the world using voiced breathing.

JOINED BREATHING

Relax in a comfortable position with your partner so that both of you can place your hands over the baby. This quiet communication through touch and breathing generates harmony between the three of you, now and in years to come. Under the gentle pressure of four hands, your breathing can deepen around the birthing muscles without tensing any other muscles unnecessarily.

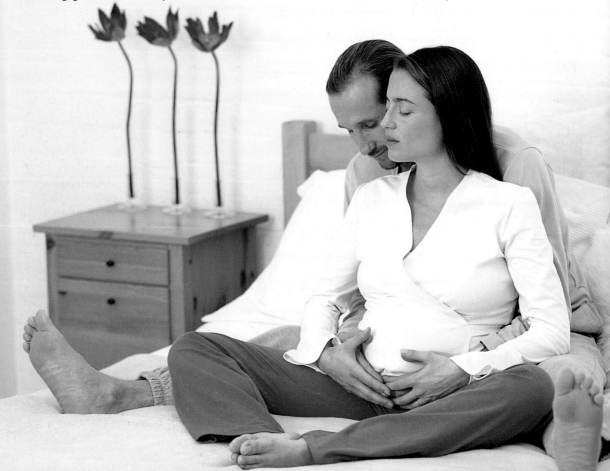

VOICED BREATHING

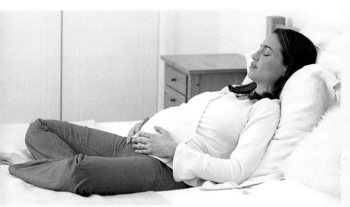

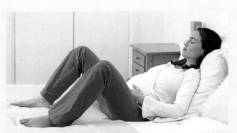

ADVANCED MOVE

Relax in a semi-reclined position with knees bent and feet hip-width apart. Target different muscles using voiced breathing as if you are ready to give birth. A deep, grunting "Huuh" activates the muscles of the perineum that move the baby down the birth canal; "Hooh" activates the muscles around the uterus.

Relax on a bed in a semi-reclined position with your legs resting comfortably. Inhale and breathe out making a long sound. This may be an "Aaah" sound, or a sound you make without opening your mouth. Use either method to explore different sounds until you can feel strong vibrations beneath your hands while remaining relaxed.

VISUALIZATION

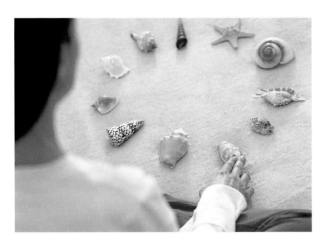

Any positive visualization experience you can practise may be a great help during labour. Choose familiar objects that specially appeal to you and arrange them in a circular pattern. Slowly retrace this pattern either physically, using your hand, or mentally. This simple yet effective technique will help to occupy your mind during contractions.

DRAWING INWARDS

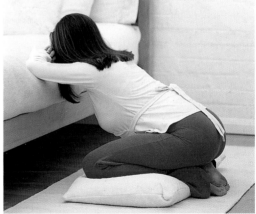

Practise "drawing inwards" to synchronize your breathing with uterine contractions during labour and while bearing down. Kneel on two cushions with your knees wide apart and your head and elbows resting against a support. Exhale to release tension each time a contraction starts and ends.

YOGA FOR LABOUR

As you approach your due date, practise yoga poses for labour. Every birth is unique and labour is unpredictable, but it is becoming widely recognised that there are many benefits if mothers can move freely during labour: upright positions may reduce pain and help you to be more in control; contractions are more effective; the blood supply to the baby is improved; and the downward force of gravity while you are in a wide pelvic position means an easier birth for your baby.

STANDING HIP ROLLS

Stand a short distance from a wall. Lean forwards and push against the wall with your hands. Roll your hips slowly in a circular motion, or swing your hips from side to side, to the rhythm of your own breathing.

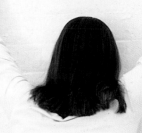

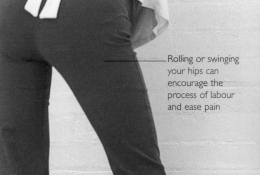

Rolling or swinging your hips can encourage the process of labour and ease pain

SUPPORTED TREE STRETCH

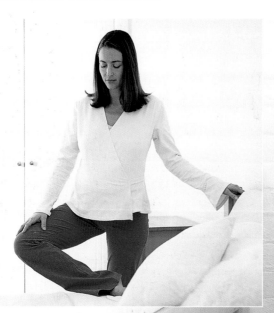

Stand in front of a low bed or a chair. Bend your left leg slightly. Inhale, lift your right knee out to the side and rest the top of your right foot on the bed. Exhale and feel the pull of gravity. Rock your pelvis gently to soothe your lower back. Repeat on the other side.

SITTING HIP ROLLS

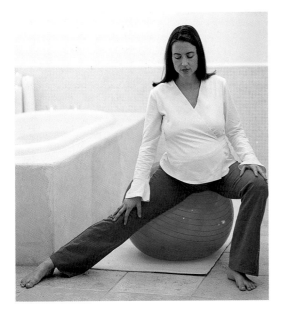

Sit on a gym ball or a low chair and sway or roll your hips in a rhythm that you find most soothing. Press your feet down and lean forwards to breathe through each contraction. Relax your shoulders with each exhalation.

ROCKING CAT

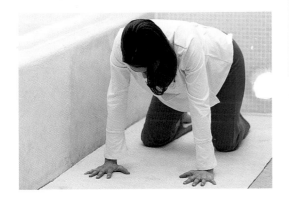

Position yourself in a strong Cat pose (p.67) with a back flat. Relax your head and gently rock your lower back to and fro to ease the pain. Press your hands down as you breathe through contractions.

SUPPORTED SQUAT

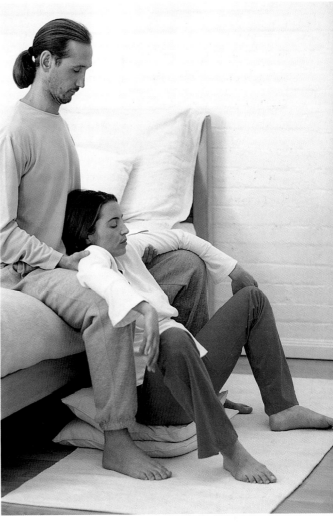

Try this position when your baby is ready to enter the world. Ask your partner to sit on a bed or a chair with his legs apart and his back straight. Place two cushions on the floor and, with your partner supporting you under your arms, drop into a wide squat between your partner's knees. Adjust the position of your feet so that your body is straight yet relaxed. Sitting on a birthing stool is also possible in this position. Practise exhaling down slowly towards your perineum.

SPECIAL APPLICATIONS

In the last weeks of pregnancy, hormonal changes may bring unexpected discomforts – even though you may be altogether fit and well. Chronic lower backache and pelvic pain may intensify due to the loosening of ligaments prior to labour and the increased weight you are carrying. The sleeplessness, heartburn and anxiety you might have experienced in the early weeks of pregnancy may well reappear. Applying yoga techniques calmly and systematically to alleviate these discomforts will help you to relax better and remain in high spirits as you prepare for labour.

PELVIC PAIN

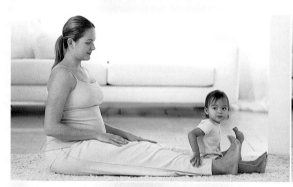 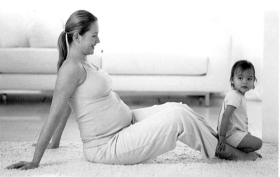

Practise this exercise after standing and walking, and particularly if you have to carry a toddler. Sit tall on the floor with straight legs. Stretch one leg forwards, then the other, as if walking on your sitting bones. Then stretch backwards, keeping your back straight.

Breathe normally. Lean back on your hands and bend your knees until you find a position in which you can move your pelvic floor muscles freely without tensing your lower abdominal muscles. Take four deep breaths, activating all these muscles with long out-breaths.

SCIATIC PAIN

Practise this exercise as often as possible to relieve pressure on your sciatic nerve. Position yourself on all fours, lower your leg on the inflamed side and let it trail limply on the floor behind you. Feel your hip drop from the waist and shake your leg until it feels floppy and relaxed.

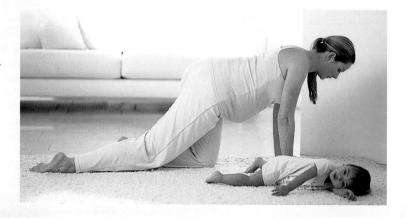

OPTIMAL FETAL POSITION

Kneel on the floor with a cushion under each knee and lean forwards onto a bed or a chair. Bring one leg out to the side and place your foot on the floor to create a strong but comfortable stretch across the base of your body. Sway your pelvis gently from side to side in this position, changing legs every few minutes. As you breathe through contractions, be aware of the pressure of your baby's head: adjust your position to increase this pressure and to facilitate your baby's optimal positioning for journeying out into the world.

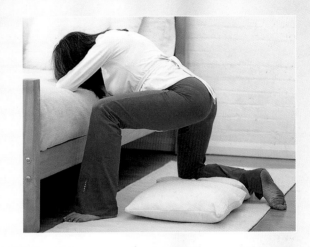

SLEEPLESSNESS

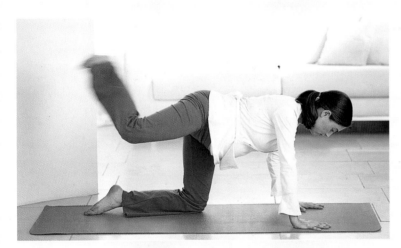

1 Leg exercises can help you to sleep better or go back to sleep if you wake in the night. Position yourself on all fours in Cat pose with your back straight, lift one knee out behind you and extend your lower leg out with a loose kick. Keep your head relaxed as you repeat this action several times on each side.

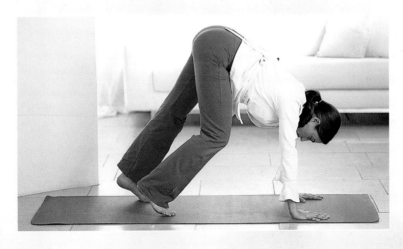

2 Sway forwards and backwards on all fours, breathing deeply. If you feel energetic enough, turn your toes under and move into Dog pose *(p.45)*, keeping your head down. Bend your knees as you walk your feet towards your hands and walk them back again. Rest in Child's pose *(p.25)* for a few minutes before standing up slowly.

NECK ROLL

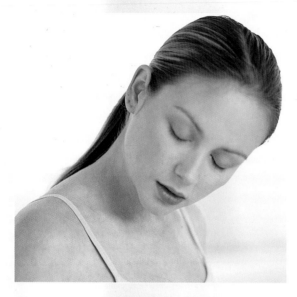

COOLING BREATH Sitakari Pranayama

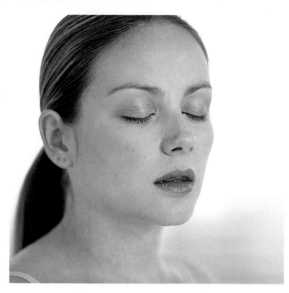

Sit up straight in a comfortable position and inhale. As you exhale, drop your chin and slowly turn your neck to the right. Relax your lower jaw. Inhale, bring your head to the centre and turn to the left as you exhale. This helps you to relax your perineum so that uterine contractions are more effective during labour.

Most women breathe through their mouth in late pregnancy. Sucking in the air with your tongue between your teeth during labour produces a pleasant cooling effect in your mouth. This practice will refresh you, particularly when contractions come fast and furious and you must pace your breathing to remain centred.

VOCAL POWER

During labour, breathing-out sounds will help to ease pain and to strengthen and lengthen your out-breath when you are required to do so. Blowing out as gently as a purring cat, for example, disengages your breath from overwhelming contractions and so avoids straining and tearing as your baby's head "crowns" through the birth canal. Sit up straight, keep your throat open and relaxed and let a sound come by itself as you breathe out.

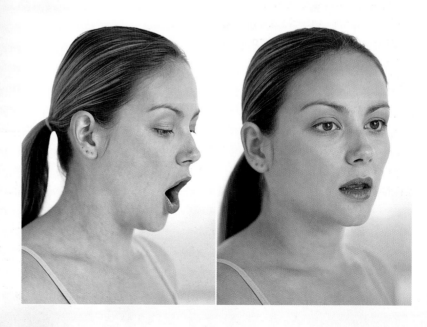

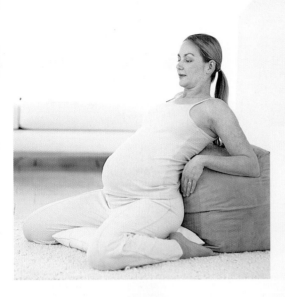

HEARTBURN

Kneel back against a pouffe, a firm beanbag or a sofa to stretch your upper body and relieve heartburn. Your lower and middle spine must be well supported so that you remain upright. Place a cushion under your buttocks, keep your knees apart, rest your weight on your elbows and take ten deep breaths.

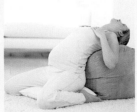

ADVANCED MOVE

If you have a firm support under your shoulder blades and you enjoy relaxing your head back, lean right back and breathe more deeply.

MEDITATION

Whether you are experienced or not in yoga, meditation may come easily to you in labour. Being able to relax and surf strong waves of contractions that bring the most acute pain is preferable to resisting and being engulfed by them. By focusing on your breathing and letting go of fear, you can access a quiet space in which you remain connected with your baby and your loved ones through the birthing process. Repeat the simple mantra, So Ham (I am That), as you breathe in and out to maintain a clear focus.

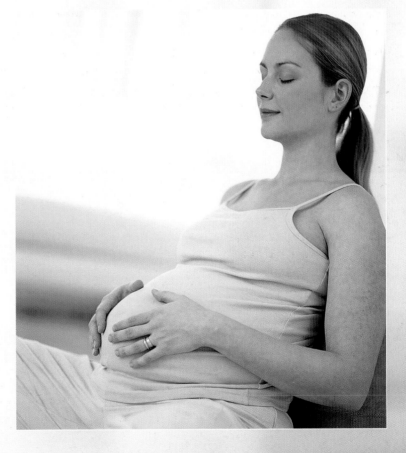

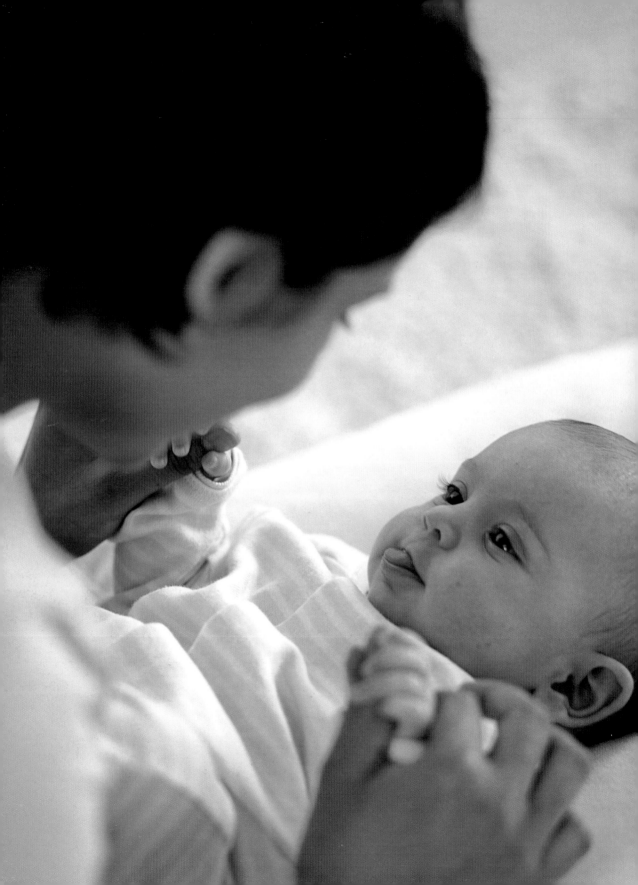

POSTNATAL
YOGA

BIRTH TO 16 WEEKS

Your life is transformed with a newborn baby, often in unexpected ways. The experience of giving birth calls for a new integration of your physical and spiritual well-being, so gentle yoga-based movements with your baby can help you, gradually and safely, to recover not only your figure and your muscle tone, but your strength from within. The flow of your breath in yoga and the stillness of deep relaxation with your baby can open up a steady, calm path ahead in the midst of all the emotions that new mothers inevitably go through.

"Little one, I embrace your presence in my life, my togetherness with you.
When were you not a part of my life and heart?"
Berber lullaby

0–6 WEEKS

For the first six weeks after giving birth, your priority is to realign your spine and strengthen your pelvic muscles. This is best done with short, simple yoga routines that can be fitted in when convenient through the day. Rest is the foundation of you and your newborn's well-being, so even if you feel fit and energetic, resist doing too much too soon. The yoga breathing and relaxation will nurture you as you nurture your baby.

COMFORTABLE BREASTFEEDING

No sooner have you welcomed your baby into the world than feeding becomes an all-absorbing task. Relaxing in a comfortable position can make a significant difference to your early experience of breastfeeding by making it more enjoyable from the start. (If you are bottle-feeding, both relaxation and yoga breath awareness while feeding can help to create a closer physical bond with your baby.)

RECLINED FEEDING

Your back should always be well supported when you breastfeed, so lie on one side with a cushion under or between your knees to make your lower back more comfortable. Place a pillow under your head to keep your shoulder on the feeding side as free as possible. If needed, raise your baby on a pillow. If you had a traumatic birth experience or a Caesarean section, lying down with your baby at your side may be the most comfortable feeding position in the weeks following the birth.

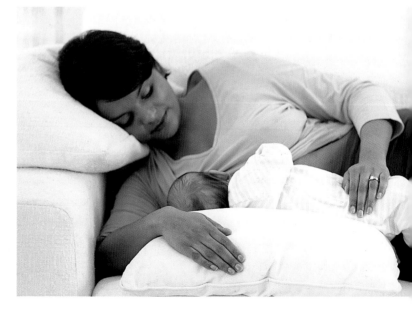

SHOULDER ROLLS

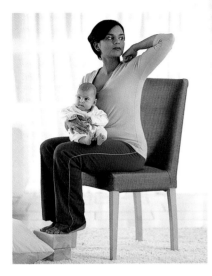

Alleviate any stiffness in your back or shoulders by sitting up straight with your back supported. Hold your baby with your right hand and place the knuckles of your left hand on your left shoulder. Breathe slowly and circle your elbow. Repeat on the other side.

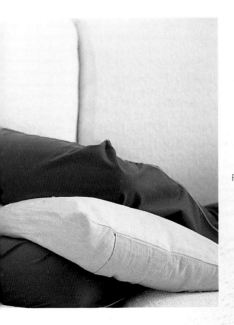

FEEDING RELAXATION

Once you are settled in a comfortable feeding position with your back aligned and your knees level with your hips, exhale deeply to release any tension. Continue this practice as your baby latches on. Keep your shoulders back and slow your breathing down to relax while remaining aware of your breath. If your baby is fretful and does not feed easily, calmly start again.

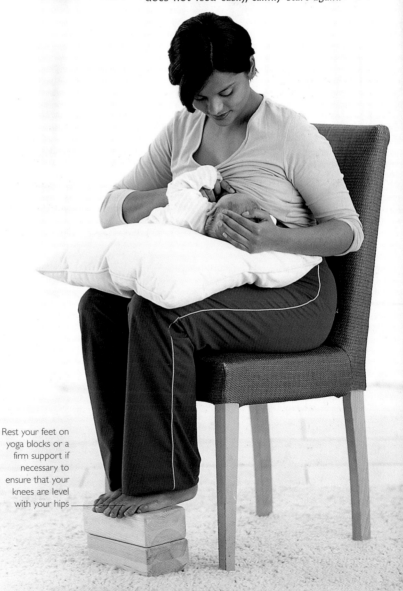

Rest your feet on yoga blocks or a firm support if necessary to ensure that your knees are level with your hips

ABDOMINAL STRETCHES
Jathara Parivartanasana

After your baby has been born, lying flat on your back again on the floor not only feels good, but is the first, safest and best way to realign your spine and use deep breathing to tone your lower back and abdominal muscles. As your uterus returns to its normal pear-sized state, all the layers of muscles around it must be strengthened to hold it in place again. Try these exercises individually or as a sequence, with or without holding your baby.

> **CAUTIONS** Ensure that:
> • Your back is aligned on the floor for Reverse breathing in order to receive the maximum benefit as you tone your pelvic floor muscles.
> • If you have had a Caesarean section, you do not practise advanced Reverse breathing.

REVERSE BREATHING

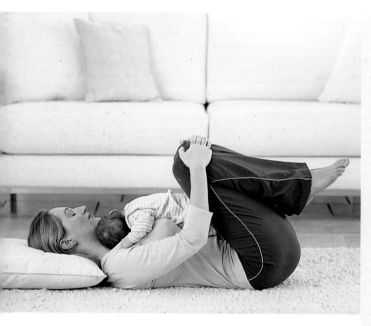

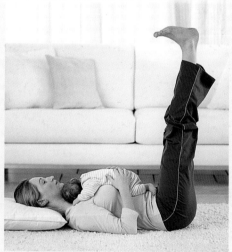

Lie on your back with a cushion under your neck and with your hands clasping your bent knees. If you are doing yoga with your baby, rest him on his tummy across your chest. Breathe deeply in your abdomen, pulling your abdominal muscles inwards and upwards as you exhale. After a week, start to draw your pelvic floor muscles up, then even further up, at the end of each exhalation.

ADVANCED MOVE
If you can lift your feet towards the ceiling with your knees bent — or, even better, with your legs straight — while remaining relaxed and comfortable, practise Reverse breathing and pull up your pelvic floor muscles while in this position. If you feel any tension, bend your knees and bring your legs down.

BACK STRENGTHENER

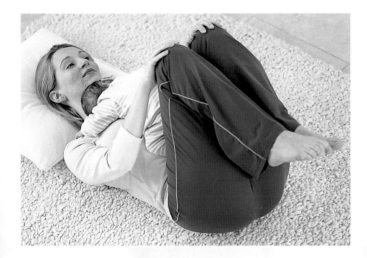

Lie on the floor with your knees bent. Place your hands gently on your knees and inhale. As you breathe out, pull your knees closer towards your chest. This action draws your waist down towards the floor and widens your upper back. If this is easy for you to do, gently move your bent knees with your hands in a clockwise, then anti-clockwise, circle. Repeat six times.

ROLL & TWIST

Lie on your back with your knees bent. Cross your arms loosely over your chest, lift your knees slightly and let yourself roll gently onto your right side on the small of your back. Try to keep your knees together. If you have had a Caesarean section, keep your knees apart and lift one knee at a time. If you are fit and want to do more, extend your left arm along the floor in a gentle twist. Breathe deeply, relax your shoulders and feel your upper back widening. Repeat several times on each side. *If you find it difficult to keep your legs and feet parallel as you roll down to the floor, let your knees move apart as you roll to the other side.*

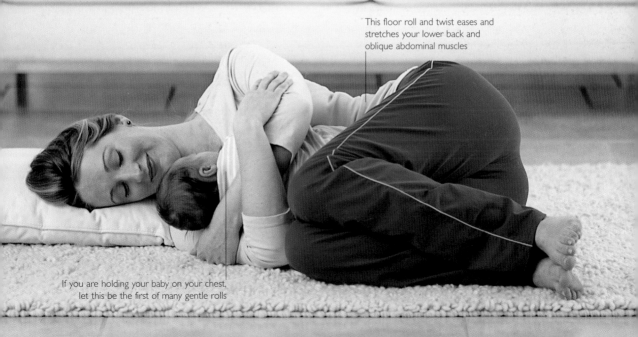

This floor roll and twist eases and stretches your lower back and oblique abdominal muscles

If you are holding your baby on your chest, let this be the first of many gentle rolls

GENTLE BACK STRETCHES

These stretches tone your dorsal muscles, which supported your baby during pregnancy. Enjoy regaining ownership of the space where your baby once was, sealing it with your yoga breathing while you remain relaxed. As you breathe from the pelvis or lower back, you also regain your physical and inner strength, realign your back, and achieve in-depth toning – all with minimal effort.

> **BENEFITS** All poses are suitable if you have had a Caesarean section. They are most effective if you:
> • Relax completely.
> • Use deep abdominal breathing.
> • Keep one or both knees bent at all times to protect your lower back.

ALIGNED POSE

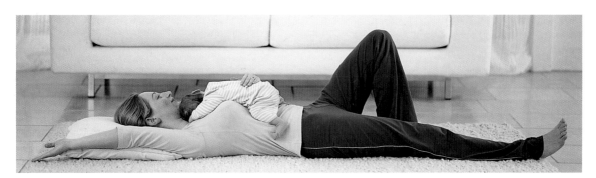

Lie on your back with a cushion under your head and your baby lying on your chest if you are doing yoga together. Bend your left knee and extend your right leg. Inhale and stretch your right arm along the floor behind your head. As you exhale, deepen the stretch from heel to fingertips. Repeat on the other side.

GENTLE TWIST

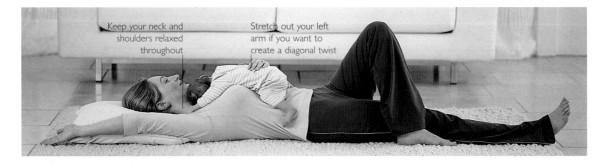

Keep your neck and shoulders relaxed throughout

Stretch out your left arm if you want to create a diagonal twist

Lie in the same position, but with your left leg crossed over your right leg. If possible, press the whole sole of your left foot on the floor. This gentle twist tones the transverse abdominal muscles. Take four deep breaths, stretching more deeply as you breathe out. Relax at the end of each exhalation. Repeat on the other side.

PRAYER POSE STRETCH

Lie on your back with your head supported, your knees bent and your feet flat on the floor. Align your spine from the base of your neck to your tail bone. Enjoy spreading your whole back flat on the floor as you breathe freely in your abdomen. Now join your palms together above your heart in Prayer pose. Inhale and press on the base of your palms as you breathe out slowly. Repeat four times, then relax.

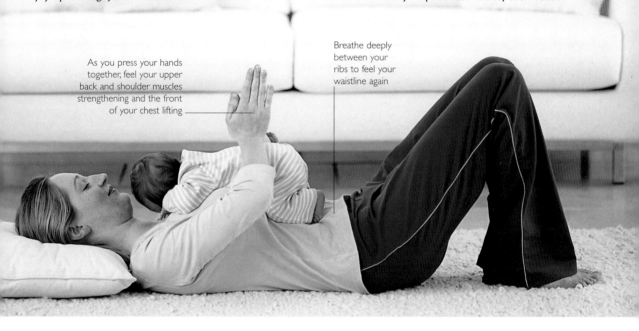

As you press your hands together, feel your upper back and shoulder muscles strengthening and the front of your chest lifting

Breathe deeply between your ribs to feel your waistline again

SELF-HUGGING STRETCH

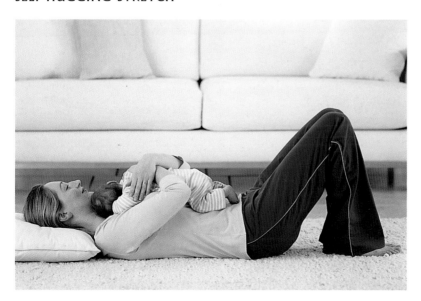

As you lie on your back with your knees bent, fold your arms across your chest. Hug yourself, and your baby too if you are holding him. Breathe deeply, feeling an expansion in your back. As you exhale, bring your shoulders and elbows down and press the base of your spine on the floor. Let your breathing realign your upper back as you remain relaxed throughout. Breathe for four cycles.

SITTING TWISTS
Bharadvajasana

These twists are a powerful way to tone and firm your body from the inside out around the waist and abdominal area. As with all yoga stretches, your breathing guides the extent of the stretch: on each out-breath, relax in your upright position and feel the expansion that allows you to twist a little further without forcing or tensing your body. Each twist should start from the base of the spine, first involving the lumbar region and then progressively the whole back.

BENEFITS Sitting twists help to:
• Combat postnatal fatigue and backache linked to poor posture.
• Strengthen the lower back muscles needed to carry larger babies and toddlers later on.
• Tone the abdominal muscles.
• Promote blood circulation in the pelvis around a Caesarean scar.

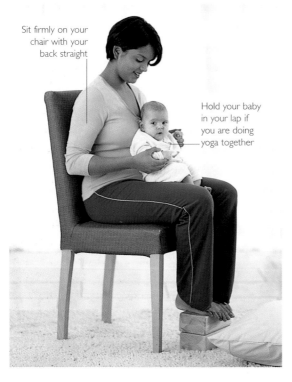

Sit firmly on your chair with your back straight

Hold your baby in your lap if you are doing yoga together

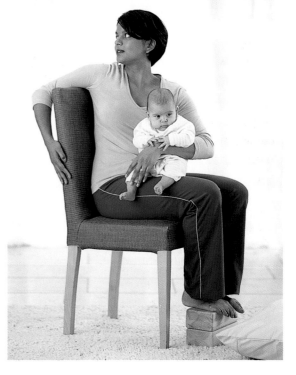

1 Sit aligned on a chair with a straight back. Support your feet if needed so that your knees are level with your hips. Keep your knees and feet together. Breathe deeply for four breaths. On each out-breath, lift your lower spine and relax your shoulders and neck.

2 Turn to the right and lift your right arm over the back of the chair. Press your sitting bones down as you progressively twist further with each exhalation for four breaths. Relax your shoulders and let your head follow the twist of your spine to the right.

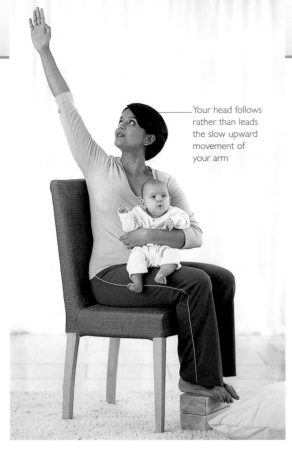

Your head follows rather than leads the slow upward movement of your arm

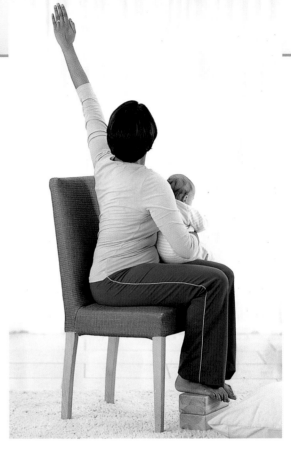

3 Breathing deeply, extend your right arm above your head. Make a slow, circling movement with your arm as you breathe in and out for one cycle. Repeat four times. Follow your hand with your eyes as you move your arm in this open twist.

4 Rest your baby on your left thigh with your right arm in a relaxed hold. *Alternatively, place the back of your right hand outside your left thigh if you are doing yoga alone.* Breathe deeply and extend your left arm above your head. Circle your arm slowly four times.

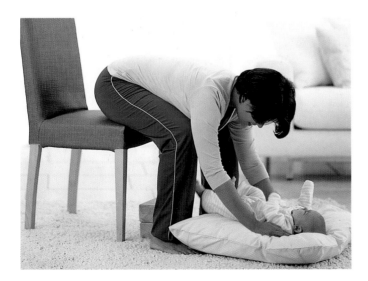

5 Ease your lower back by flopping forwards as you exhale to completely relax in a Forward bend. Extend your arms forwards to rest your baby on a cushion. You can also use this method to lower your baby to the floor after each feed.

WORK IN THE POSE

Correct twisting from the base of the spine requires a careful alignment of hips, knees and feet. Learning to let a stretch deepen with each out-breath rather than forcing it is an essential aspect of Sitting twists.

KNEELING STRETCHES

Make this short sequence your first mini workout after the birth of your baby. It enables you to stretch your body to gain stamina and lift your spirits. It also allows for a full back stretch without any strain to the abdominal muscles. The kneeling position, which you used during pregnancy, continues to create a solid base for you to stretch while close to the ground. This is an ideal sequence to prepare you for future floor play with a crawling baby.

> **BENEFITS** These stretches prevent or relieve lower backache, especially if linked to muscular tension around the sciatic nerve. They are also recommended for:
> • Women with a Caesarean scar.
> • Women who have given birth to twins or who have "split" their right abdominal muscles.

UPPER BODY STRETCH

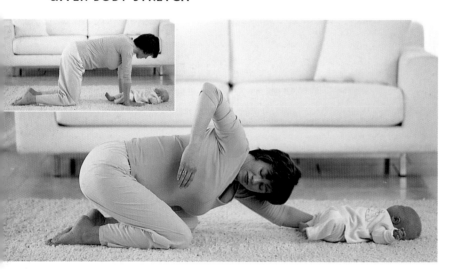

1 Position yourself on all fours with your baby resting on a comfortable surface near you. Sit back on your heels to stretch your arms, then bend your right elbow to open your chest fully. Rotate your shoulder in a circular movement. Breathe in and out four times as you circle your bent arm. Rest if you feel tired.

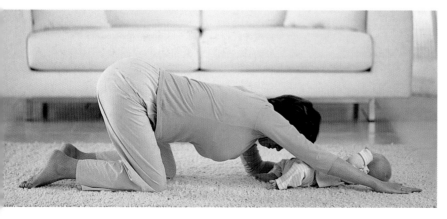

2 Stretch your right arm forwards as far as you can. Use your left forearm as a support so that you can extend into your fingers. At the same time, extend your tail bone back towards your heels. Breathe deeply four times, then return to an all-fours position.

FULL BACK STRETCH

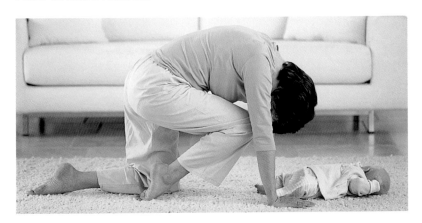

1 Begin on all fours with your back flat. Inhale, relax your head and lift your shoulders in Cat pose (p.67). On your next in-breath bring one knee towards your head, keeping your calf muscle and foot relaxed. Relax your knee down as you breathe out. Alternate each leg to achieve a full stretch of your spine.

2 From Cat pose, bring one knee towards your head as you inhale, then exhale and extend that leg out behind you. Keep your leg relaxed from the hip. Relax your head and allow a full extension of your body in a straight line from shoulders to heel. Repeat on the other side.

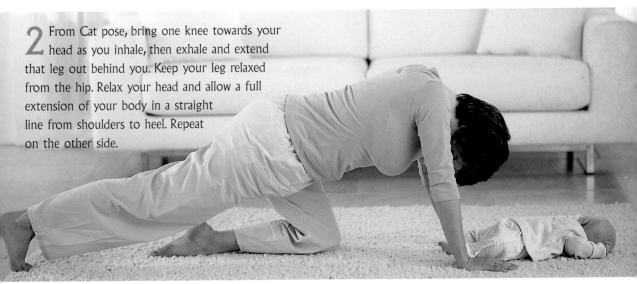

RESTING POSE

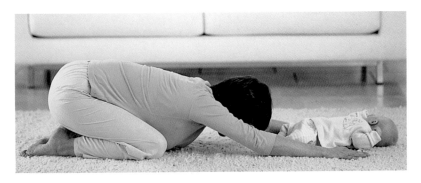

Relax in Swan pose by sitting back on your heels with your arms relaxed and outstretched in front of you on the floor. *Alternatively, rest on your forearms if this feels more comfortable.* Press your hands down as you exhale and relax your head completely.

RELAXATION

Deep rest and relaxation after childbirth are not given enough priority in the West. It is therefore important that you make time to relax in the weeks after your baby is born, whatever your lifestyle. Including your baby in your relaxation from day one is very rewarding as he will learn to enjoy this calm state too. Use these techniques whenever you can through the day to renew your energy, nurture yourself as a mother and pacify your baby.

> **BENEFITS** Mixed emotions such as anger and sadness are normal at this time as you undergo hormonal changes. Relaxation helps you to:
> • Acknowledge and surrender feelings of tiredness.
> • Overcome any anxiety that you may not be a good enough mother.
> • Avoid a build-up of tension.

CONSCIOUS SURRENDER

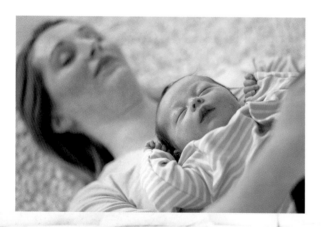

Lie flat on the floor or a bed with your baby on your chest. Make sure you are both comfortable, then breathe freely and quieten your body and mind in stillness. With each out-breath, voiced as an "Aaah" sound if you wish, release tension. Breathe gently in and out with awareness for a few moments, consciously surrendering to the wonder of your baby's new life.

CORPSE POSE WITH BABY

Lie on your back on the floor with your knees bent to protect your lower back. Place a pillow under your neck and rest your baby on his tummy across your chest. Once you are both settled and comfortable, avoid further movements. Close your eyes and let go to access a state of deep rest that soothes your nervous system.

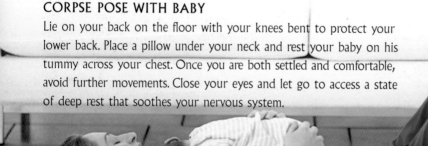

INSTANT MEDITATION

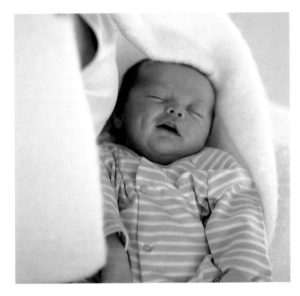

After you have fed your baby, or if your baby has just fallen asleep in your arms, take a moment to stop and relax. Empty your mind of the many tasks that need to be done, as they can wait while you absorb yourself in the present. The more regular your practice, the more effective and enjoyable it will be.

PACIFYING

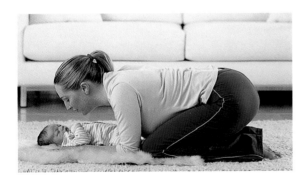

If you do not know why your baby is crying, gentle humming or singing helps you to release tension and lengthen your out-breaths. An all-fours position may be a comfortable way to relax by your baby if you used it while pregnant, or if your back is sore.

WALKING RELAXATION

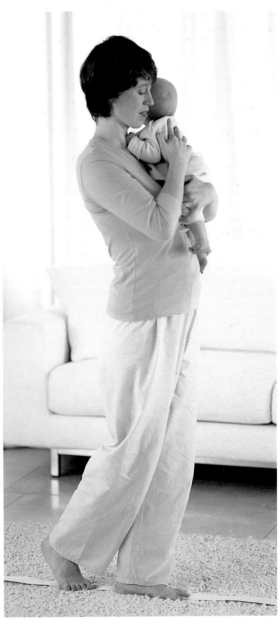

Hold your baby with your spine erect and your weight evenly distributed. Keep your knees slightly bent to ensure spinal alignment. Walk with very small steps, breathing freely, along a line or in a circle. Let go of any thoughts or emotions with each step you take.

6–16 WEEKS

Let your progression towards more dynamic yoga be guided by your needs: you may wish to continue practising relaxed stretches close to the floor; or move onto more vigorous limbering sequences. Pace yourself, watch the flow of your breath in your movements and always relax afterwards. If your baby needs your attention in the middle of a sequence, return to your starting position and exhale to relax. Then smile and greet your baby.

STANDING TALL

Standing tall refers not only to having a straight back, but to using your pelvic floor, abdominal muscles and lower back muscles to hold your pelvis in perfect alignment with your spine. It is only while in this aligned Mountain pose that stretching becomes truly beneficial. Having aligned yourself against the wall to monitor your spinal curves when pregnant, this can now become an enjoyable practice with your baby.

SPINAL ALIGNMENT

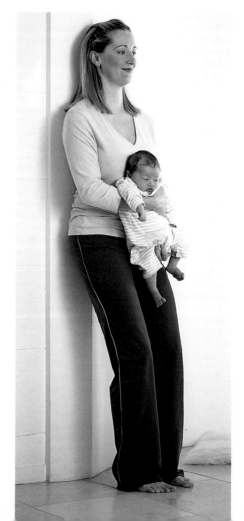

CAUTION The distance of your feet from the wall depends on your spinal curve. Start with a distance at which your back is comfortable before gradually moving your feet closer to the wall as your alignment improves. If needed, place a cushion between your middle back and the wall to begin with. Practise first without your baby to concentrate on your breathing. Only practise the advanced move if you are confident holding your baby in a relaxed way.

Stand a short distance from a wall with your knees bent loosely and your baby in your arms. Align the length of your spine against the wall. Pull your abdominal muscles up as you inhale, and open your chest as you exhale. Lower your chin and lengthen the back of your neck. As your alignment improves, stand closer to the wall.

OPTIONAL PELVIC FLOOR LIFT

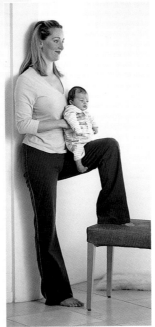

If you have had a Caesarean section, or your baby does not like being lifted up in the air at present, place one foot on a chair or stool. Hold your baby on your raised leg with a relaxed hold. As you press your back against the wall, practise Reverse breathing (p.128) slowly, lengthening each out-breath before releasing your pelvic floor at the end of the exhalation. Repeat with the other leg.

PELVIC FLOOR LIFT

Use the rhythm of your breathing to lift your pelvic floor as part of your spinal realignment while playing with your baby. Raise your baby slowly in the air above your head as you inhale and lift your pelvic floor muscles. Lower your baby gently as you exhale and continue to lift your pelvic floor muscles. Release them at the end of the out-breath. Repeat three times if your baby is happy.

ADVANCED MOVE

Place your left foot on your right knee. Align your left knee and hip to elongate your spine and correct the tilt of your pelvis. Hold your baby safely yet loosely on your left thigh. Exhale and raise your right arm up against the wall. Take four deep breaths. Lift your pelvic floor muscles as you inhale. Press your shoulder against the wall with each exhalation. Repeat on the other side.

KNEELING SUN SALUTATION

If you are not yet ready for the exertion of dynamic standing poses, this adapted Sun salutation allows you to experience a full stretch while remaining grounded as you move in and out of an all-fours position. Take your time and progress gently from one pose to the next, relaxing in between each move. With practice, aim to repeat this sequence twice on each side every day in a flowing motion that is guided by the rhythm of your breathing.

BENEFITS Having turned your hips and knees out through the many weeks of pregnancy, this sequence takes you back to the alignment and symmetry of classic yoga to centre and strengthen you. These balancing poses will also help you to regain your agility.

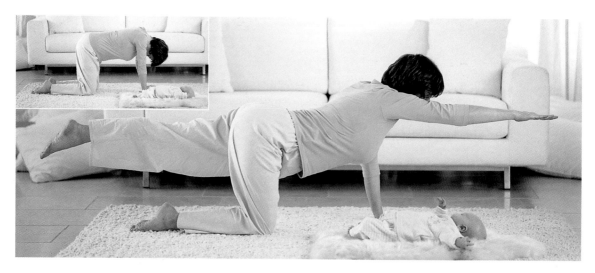

1 Place your baby in a safe position near you. Move into a well aligned all-fours position with your knees directly under your hips and your hands under your shoulders. Align your neck and spine.

As you inhale, raise your right arm and your left leg to create a strong line from hand to foot. As you exhale, stretch further through your wrists to your fingertips and through your knee to your heel.

2 Exhale and lower your arm. On your next out-breath, bend your extended leg, move it forwards and place your foot between your hands. Stretch your lower spine and keep your hips aligned as you press down firmly with your left foot to prevent your knee turning out.

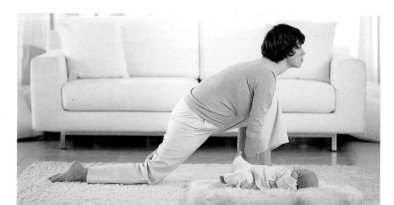

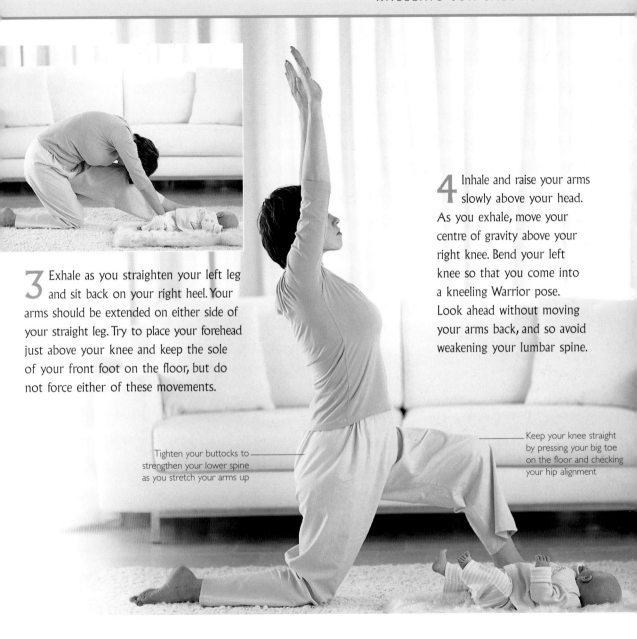

3 Exhale as you straighten your left leg and sit back on your right heel. Your arms should be extended on either side of your straight leg. Try to place your forehead just above your knee and keep the sole of your front foot on the floor, but do not force either of these movements.

4 Inhale and raise your arms slowly above your head. As you exhale, move your centre of gravity above your right knee. Bend your left knee so that you come into a kneeling Warrior pose. Look ahead without moving your arms back, and so avoid weakening your lumbar spine.

Tighten your buttocks to strengthen your lower spine as you stretch your arms up

Keep your knee straight by pressing your big toe on the floor and checking your hip alignment

5 Inhale, and on your next out-breath lower your arms and place your left knee on the floor in line with your right knee. Slowly sit back on your heels in Swan pose with your arms extended in front of you. *Alternatively, relax in Child's pose with your arms turned out on each side of your body.*

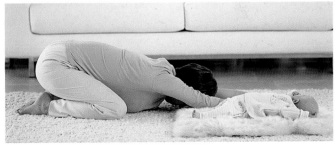

STANDING SUN SALUTATION

This adapted postnatal Sun salutation increases your strength and stamina while preparing you to move into, or resume, more classic yoga poses. Without discontinuing your relaxed stretches on the floor, the time may now be right for you to expand these gentle movements into a regular practice of postures that increase your energy and enjoyment of life, day by day. Ensure that you remain centred and balanced with your baby in this new vitality.

BENEFITS Use this flowing sequence of stretches and Forward bends to move gracefully and easily, keeping an uplift in your lower back at all times. Proceed at your own pace, practising one pose at a time and relaxing between steps at first if this approach feels easier.

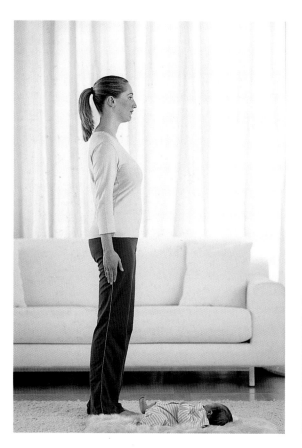

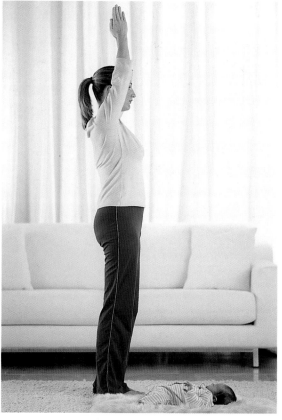

1 Place your baby in a safe position near you. Stand tall in a steady Mountain pose with your feet only slightly apart and your arms straight at your sides. Breathe freely and centre yourself.

2 Inhale, join your hands in Prayer pose and raise your arms above your head. Avoid arching your lower back and keep the back of your neck extended. Stretch from heels to fingertips as you breathe out.

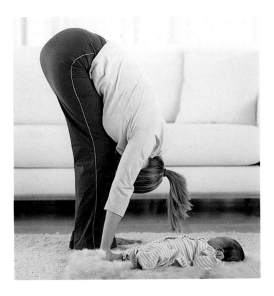

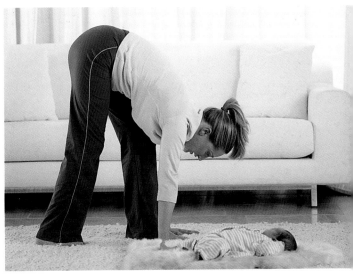

3 Keep your legs extended or slightly bent as you exhale, bend forwards and place your palms on the floor either side of your feet.

4 Keep your hands in position, and on your next in-breath begin to walk your feet three or four small steps backwards, keeping your knees bent.

5 Keep your knees slightly bent and parallel as you align your feet and stretch your back fully in Dog pose. Then straighten your legs as much as you can. Avoid turning your knees out as you did when pregnant. The base of your spine is the apex of the pose as you stretch from your hands up your back, and from your feet up your legs.

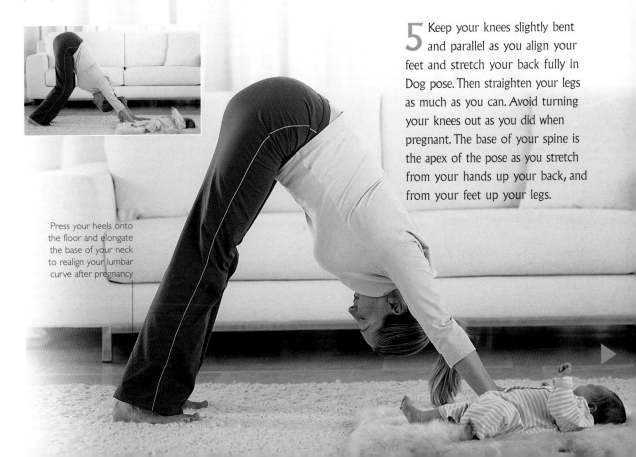

Press your heels onto the floor and elongate the base of your neck to realign your lumbar curve after pregnancy

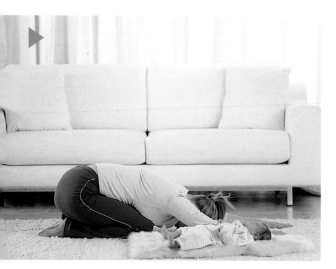

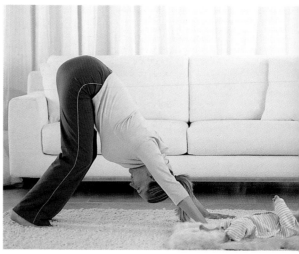

6 Keep your hands in position and bend your knees to come down into Child's pose. Relax your arms and head on the floor in this counterpose and rest for two breaths.

7 On an in-breath, come onto your toes and raise your hips up as high as possible again in Dog pose. Keep your knees slightly bent as you straighten your back.

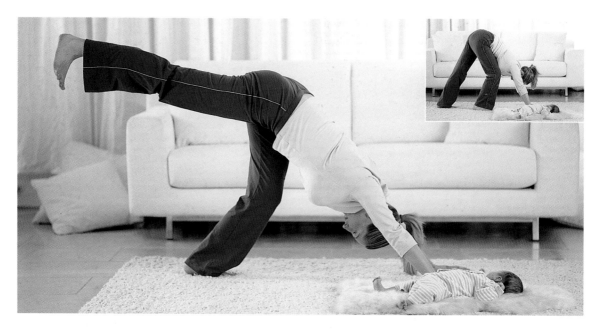

8 Inhale and extend your right leg out behind you. Keep your left leg bent and stretch into your right heel as you exhale. Lower your leg and repeat on the other side, then come onto your toes and continue stretching your back as you walk your feet slowly towards your hands. Keep your head relaxed. *If you wish, practise walking back into Dog pose and then forwards again as a separate strengthening movement.*

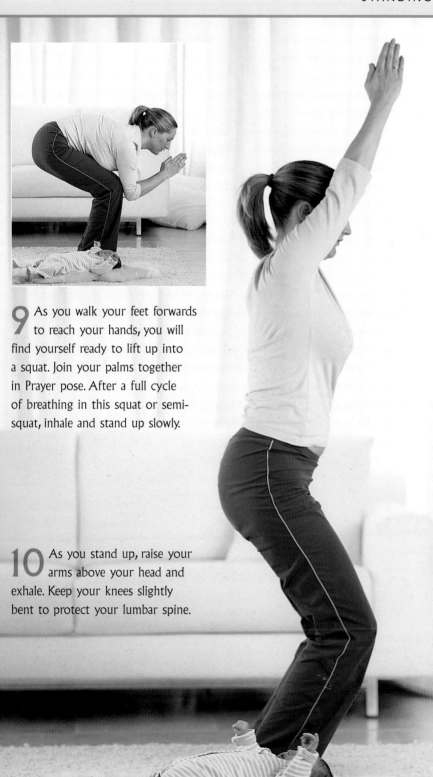

9 As you walk your feet forwards to reach your hands, you will find yourself ready to lift up into a squat. Join your palms together in Prayer pose. After a full cycle of breathing in this squat or semi-squat, inhale and stand up slowly.

10 As you stand up, raise your arms above your head and exhale. Keep your knees slightly bent to protect your lumbar spine.

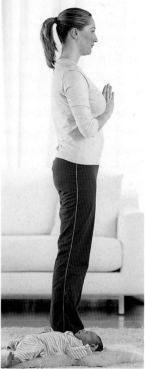

11 Inhale, straighten your legs and lower your hands to chest level. As you fix your gaze in front of you, become aware, with a centred mindfulness, of the room and of your baby lying beside you.

RELAXATION

Resuming the demands of your life as a woman, particularly if you are planning to return to work, and balancing them with mothering your growing baby requires new skills in alternating activity and rest. Draw the strength you need to face unexpected challenges from reserves of deep relaxation. A few minutes of deep rest are the best substitute for missed sleep while your baby still feeds at night, and the unconditional love of mothers for their babies can best flourish through constant resourcing in the silence and stillness of relaxation.

> **BENEFITS** A regular practice of simple relaxation helps you to:
> • Dissolve stress as it arises every day and so avoid any build-up of tension and fatigue.
> • Relax and let go, creating space for quality time with loved ones.
> • Take your time to heal a difficult birth experience or trauma, forgiving yourself and all involved.

DEEP REST

Lie comfortably on your back on the floor, or on a firm bed, so that your whole spine is aligned. Use cushions if needed under your head and knees. Rest your baby on her tummy across your abdomen, then relax your arms and hands loosely at your sides and close your eyes. As you exhale, press your back gently down, feeling totally supported. Open your eyes again, retaining this feeling, then close your eyes and relax. Exploring the threshold between alertness and full relaxation helps you to access deep rest whenever you need it. With practice, turn your palms up to achieve a softer and deeper relaxation.

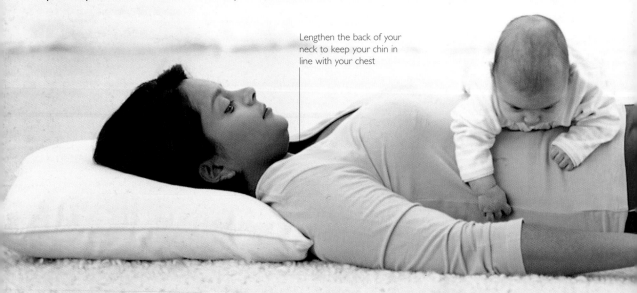

Lengthen the back of your neck to keep your chin in line with your chest

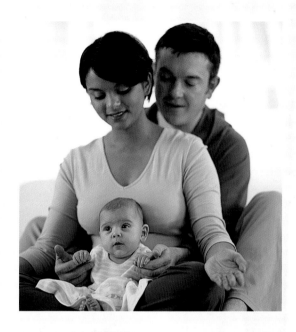

MEDITATION

Times of quietly celebrating your baby's presence are precious to nurture, and strengthen your bond with your baby. If possible, involve your partner or whoever you wish to include in this meditation. Sit cross-legged with your baby in your lap and with the backs of your hands resting on your knees. Sit your partner close behind you with his legs apart so that he can hold your baby's hands. Relax in the stillness, breathing quietly, and experience the quality of rest that results.

RELAXED FIELD

Use this joint relaxation often to let go of unwanted emotions and nurture a loving bond with your baby. Lie on your back with your knees bent and your baby supported by your thighs. Relax and let go of physical and mental tension while still being fully aware of your baby.

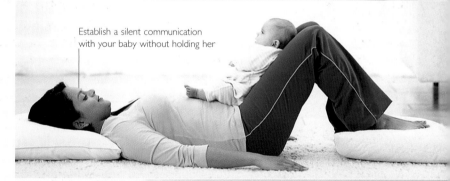

Establish a silent communication with your baby without holding her

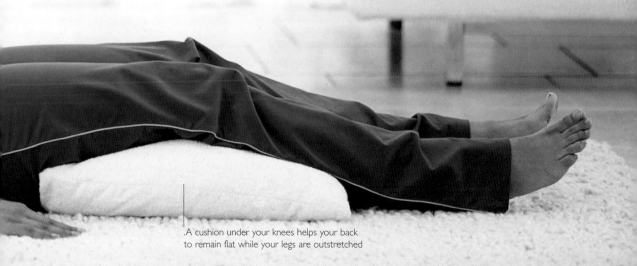

A cushion under your knees helps your back to remain flat while your legs are outstretched

STANDING FORWARD BEND
Adapted Parsvottanasana

These deceptively simple stretches using a support help you to enjoy the benefits of a fully stretched back. They also keep your shoulders supple and your chest open as you spend time cradling and feeding your baby. The open twist at the start expands your rib cage and energizes you, while the Forward bend aligns your hips and helps you to gain more extension in your lower back.

> **CAUTIONS** If Forward bends are a challenge after pregnancy:
> • Use a support that suits your physique and level of fitness – a low or high chair or a table top.
> • Practise each step separately to regain your balance gradually.

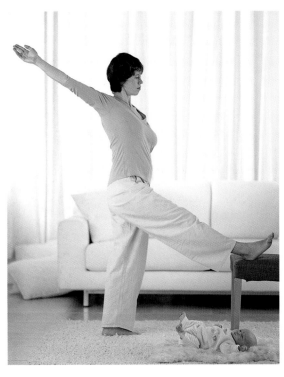

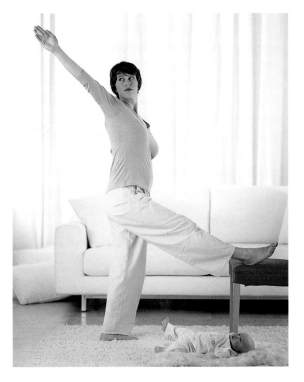

1 Lay your baby in a safe position near you. Stand in Mountain pose facing a chair or an alternative support. Make sure that when you raise your right leg, you can rest your heel comfortably on the chair seat. Face your support, raise your right arm in the air and extend it back as far as you can. Breathe deeply for four breaths.

2 Extend the stretch further by twisting your upper body round to the right and turning your head to look up at your hand. Raise your extended arm slightly higher in order to obtain the most extreme twisting action that is possible for you at this time. Breathe deeply for four breaths. Then repeat steps 1 and 2 on the left side.

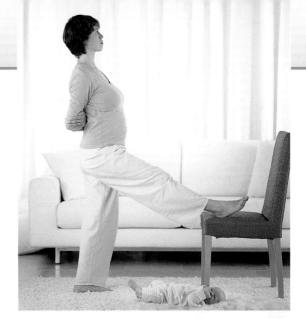

3 Place your right heel on the chair again and clasp both elbows behind your back. When you have regained a balanced and upright posture, extend your hips, waist and chest upwards, stretching both sides of your body evenly for four breaths.

4 On an out-breath, bend your torso forwards and down slowly towards your right leg. Bend your left knee slightly to ease into a Forward bend, and keep your head relaxed. Come up slowly on an in-breath. Repeat steps 3 and 4 on the left side.

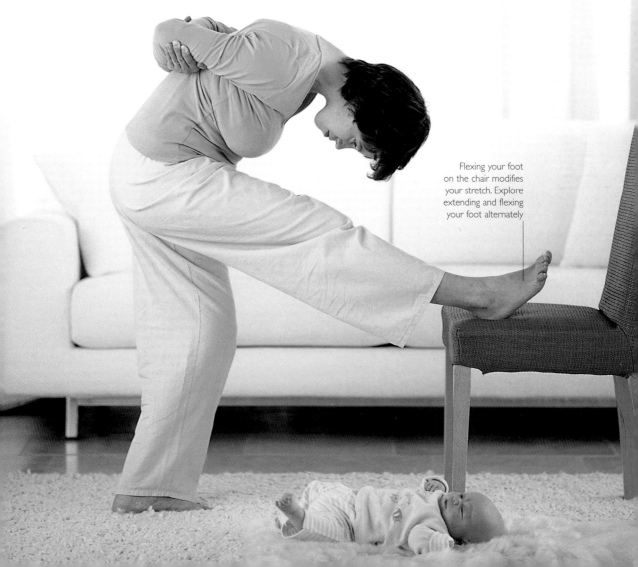

Flexing your foot on the chair modifies your stretch. Explore extending and flexing your foot alternately

TWISTS & BENDS

The increased flexibility of your hip joints due to hormonal changes in pregnancy can sometimes mask stiffness in your lower back. These sitting poses both strengthen the hips after childbirth and help to elongate your lower spine to restore strength and mobility in your back. Although you should progress slowly and gradually through these twists and bends, a regular practice (which can become a part of playing with your baby on the floor), will yield visible results within weeks. As ever in yoga, your breath is your main tool as you work through each pose.

> ### BENEFITS AND CAUTIONS
> Practising twists and bends using deep breathing not only improves the flexibility of your back, it relieves backache and promotes a healthy digestion by removing sluggishness. Twists also help to bring together "split" right abdominal muscles.
>
> If you have had a Caesarean section, gently practise Sitting twists from eight weeks after the birth.

SITTING TWISTS

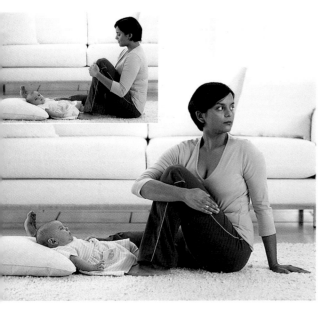

Easy twist Rest your baby on a comfortable surface near you. Sit with your right leg extended, your left knee bent and your left foot on the floor. Straighten your back and press your left hand on the floor behind you as you turn to the left and hug your left knee with your right arm. Repeat on the other side.

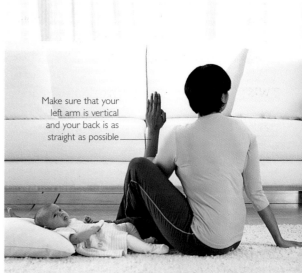

Make sure that your left arm is vertical and your back is as straight as possible

Classic twist Extend your right leg and place your left foot on the floor outside your right knee. Twist round to the right, using your right hand as a support. Press the inside of your left knee and your left elbow against each other to push your torso round for four successive exhalations. Repeat on the left side.

EASY FORWARD BEND

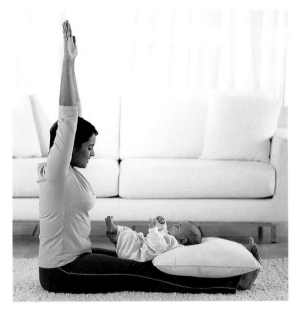

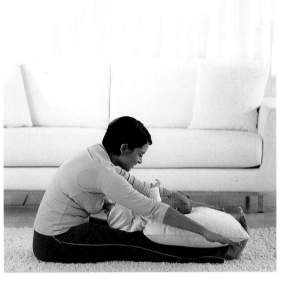

1 Sit tall, stretching from seat to crown. Extend both legs, relax your shoulders and neck and rest your baby on your legs if you are doing yoga together. Inhale, raise your arms up and exhale in the stretch.

2 On your next out-breath, lean forwards from the hips and lower your hands towards your toes. Extend the backs of your knees and relax your head as you stretch your spine for four exhalations.

TWISTING FORWARD BEND

RESTING POSE

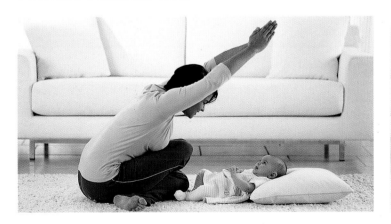

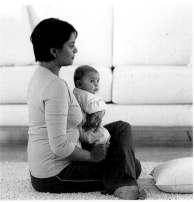

Sit tall, then cross your legs, one over the other, so that your right knee rests above your left knee. Keep your hips aligned. Raise your arms and join your palms. Breathe freely as you lean forwards with a straight back. Repeat with your legs crossed over the other way.

End these poses by sitting up straight with your legs crossed comfortably. Enjoy your newly strengthened posture as you pick up your baby.

ROLLING PLOUGH
Halasana

This stimulating floor sequence uses a rhythmical rolling movement to maximize the benefits of the Plough postnatally. As you move your spine back and forth, your roll can be as small or as acrobatic as you can, or want to, make it. Keep your body relaxed and never force a movement: if you cannot lift your feet over your head at first, just enjoy yourself and try again later.

> **CAUTIONS** If you have had a Caesarean section:
> • Do not practise this sequence until eight weeks after the birth.
> • Start by practising small rolls at first until you can roll back fully into Plough without strain.

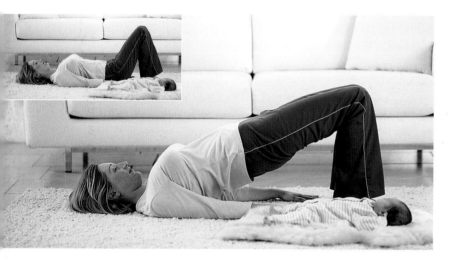

1 Lie on the floor with your legs bent, your knees together and your arms at your sides. As you breathe in, lift your pelvis off the floor, as high as feels comfortable. Keep your knees in a straight line. Grip the base of your spine with your buttock muscles and keep them tensed as you breathe out. Lift your pelvic floor up again, then relax as you breathe out.

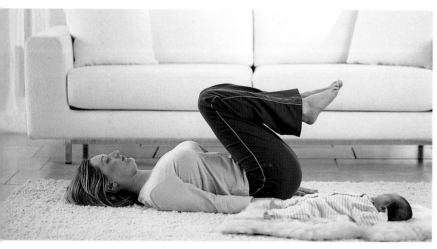

2 Breathe in, and on your next out-breath, release your buttock muscles and lower your pelvis slowly to the floor. At the same time, bring your knees as close to your chest as you can. Lengthen your spine and point your toes through two cycles of deep abdominal breathing. Repeat steps 1 and 2 three times.

3 On your next out-breath, push the palms of your hands down on the floor as you lift your hips and roll them backwards, keeping your knees bent. Let your arms follow the movement of your legs as they roll back.

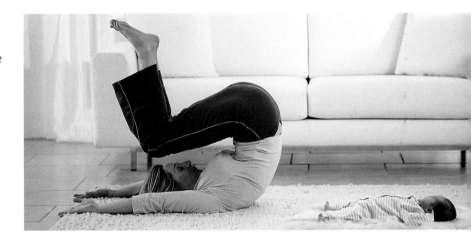

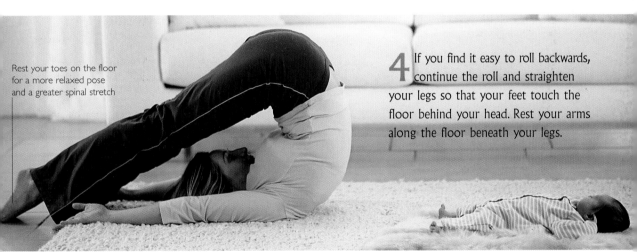

Rest your toes on the floor for a more relaxed pose and a greater spinal stretch

4 If you find it easy to roll backwards, continue the roll and straighten your legs so that your feet touch the floor behind your head. Rest your arms along the floor beneath your legs.

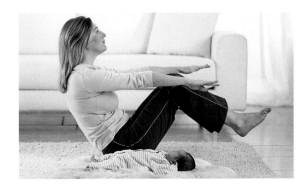

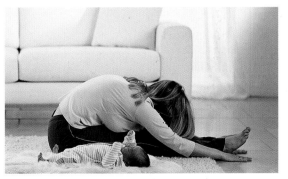

5 Inhale, bend your knees and extend your arms in front of you to ease your forward roll back up. Use momentum to stretch forwards as you exhale.

6 Continue the momentum and roll into a Sitting forward bend at the end of the exhalation. Then inhale, roll back down onto your back and relax.

SPECIAL APPLICATIONS

Rather than targeting particular problems or pain after childbirth, work through the other gentle exercises in this chapter first – they have all been carefully worked out to address hormonal imbalances, poor muscle tone and lack of sleep. They also tone your body with a perfect alignment of hips and spine because regaining good posture is a major factor in promoting a sense of well-being, now and in the long term. However, if you still experience problems, try these special applications. As always, deep breathing and relaxation in the poses are essential for success.

SPLIT MUSCLES

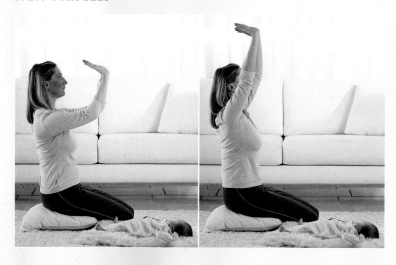

Kneel upright with your back straight and a cushion between your buttocks and feet. Practise Reverse breathing *(p.128)* by drawing your pelvic floor muscles and lower back muscles up as you inhale, then even further up as you exhale. Extend your out-breath for as long as possible before releasing it. Push your hands, palms up, in an upward movement in front of your face through four cycles of breathing.

WEAK PELVIC FLOOR

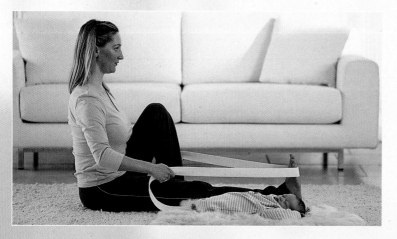

Sit tall on the floor with your right leg extended. Bend your left knee and position your foot firmly on the floor. Turn the toes of your right foot up and place a yoga belt around the ball of your foot. Drop your chin, pull evenly on either end of the belt with both hands, and draw your pelvic floor muscles up as you inhale, then even further up as you exhale. Repeat with the other leg.

CONFLICTING EMOTIONS

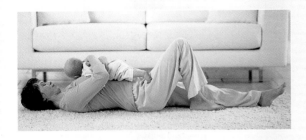

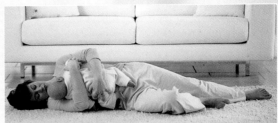

1 Acknowledge your feelings and release them without guilt: lie on your back, either alone or holding your baby across your chest, and bend your right knee.

2 Roll onto your right side, keeping your body relaxed. Bend your left leg and roll onto that side. Breathe more deeply as you roll to and fro ten times.

UPLIFTING SEQUENCE

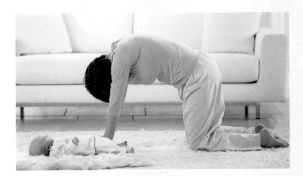

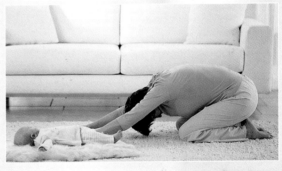

1 Start on all fours in Cat pose *(p.67)*. Arch your spine and relax your head as you breathe in. If you wish, exhale with a deep "Aaah" sound to release tension.

2 On your next out-breath, sit back on your heels without moving your hands. Keep your head low. Sit on a cushion for comfort if necessary.

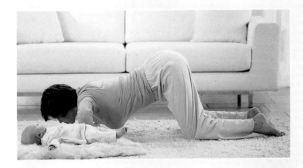

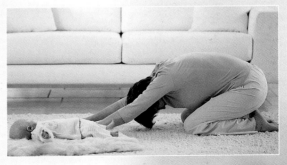

3 Inhale and stretch forwards, moving your weight onto your hands. As you reach the limit of your stretch, lift your shoulders and lower your head.

4 Exhale and lean back with an arched spine to sit on your heels again. Repeat the sequence to engage your emotions in this flow of breathing.

GLOSSARY

Abdominal breathing
Awareness of the involvement of the abdominal muscles, together with the diaphragm, in the steady rhythm of inhalations and exhalations.

Abdominal muscles
Muscles linking the rib cage to the base of the pelvis. Three main lateral muscles – transverse abdominal, and internal and external obliques – are attached to the right abdominal muscle at the front of the body.

Birthing muscles
The transverse abdominal muscle, the powerful muscular walls of the uterus and pelvic floor muscles are directly involved in your baby's journey through the pelvis during the birthing process.

Counterpose
A pose that produces effects which are opposite or complementary to a previous pose, and therefore desirable in order to achieve a balanced cycle.

Grounding
When the centre of gravity in the lower back is in harmony with the earth's downward force, the lower body from the waist down is "grounded". This promotes calm and balance.

Haemorrhoids
Varicose veins of the rectum that affect 20–50% of pregnant women. Constipation often causes or exacerbates this condition.

Heartburn
In early and late pregnancy, an increase in the production of progesterone and oestrogen relaxes smooth muscles. Heartburn occurs when the ring of muscle that separates the oesophagus from the stomach relaxes, allowing stomach acid to reflux into the oesophagus.

High blood pressure in pregnancy
If elevated blood pressure readings are accompanied by rapid weight gain, swollen joints and protein in the urine (indicating pre-eclampsia) treatment is required immediately.

Integration
Yoga poses have multiple effects on the cardiovascular, nervous, digestive and endocrine systems. These effects are best integrated during the relaxation that must follow all practice.

Inverted pose
A pose in which the pelvis is higher than the head. Inverting inner organs activates sluggish parts, brings blood to the brain and improves circulation.

Involuntary muscles
Also known as smooth muscles. They are regulated by the autonomic nervous system, so their function is completely involuntary, for example, the muscles of the uterus and the digestive tract.

Ligaments
Dense bands of connective tissue fibres that attach one bone to another.

Micro-movement
A small yet focused movement that results in a stretching of the deepest layers of muscles in the body. Stretching is effected through breathing and awareness.

Pelvic area
The pelvis is made up of four bones: the sacrum, the hip bones, and the symphysis pubis that joins the two pubic bones at the front of the pelvis. The pelvic area comprises all the pelvic ligaments and the muscles that link the pelvis to the spine, the rib cage and the legs.

Pelvic breathing
The "roots" of the diaphragm (the main muscle involved in breathing) are associated with both the lower back and pelvic muscles. This is why a correct alignment of the lower spine relieves tension in the diaphragm and promotes deeper breathing.

Prone pose
A pose that is practised with your body lying flat on its front.

Restorative yoga
The practice of relaxation, meditation, deep breathing or supported poses with the aim of nurturing or healing the body or mind with a minimum of physical and mental effort.

Reverse breathing
After giving birth, the action of toning the pelvic muscles changes. The pelvic floor muscles are lifted on an in-breath, lifted even further during the exhalation, and released only at the

end of the exhalation. This restores their elasticity and tones the transverse abdominal muscle around the uterus as it returns to its pre-pregnancy size.

Sacrum
The triangular bony structure made up of the fused lowest five vertebrae in the spinal column. Its broad surface provides an extensive area to which the muscles responsible for leg movement are attached.

Sciatica
Inflammation due to pressure on the sciatic nerve, causing lower back, buttock and leg pain. The pressure of the enlarging uterus is a common cause of sciatica in pregnancy.

SPD (Symphysis pubis dysfunction)
Separation of the lower joint of the pubic bones in the pelvis. This separation can cause severe localized pain in the pelvic area and impair mobility.

Spinal muscles
All the muscles of the trunk that extend, rotate and allow lateral flexion of the spinal column.

Split abdominal muscles
Tearing of the fascial sheath, or linea alba, that joins the two vertical muscular bands of the right abdominal muscle.

Supine pose
A pose that is practised with your body lying flat on its back.

Vena cava
The major vein delivering systemic blood to the heart.

USEFUL ADDRESSES & WEBSITES

UK

YOGA
Birthlight
P.O.Box 148, Cambridge CB4 2GB
Tel 01223 362288
www.birthlight.com
Email: enquiries@birthlight.com
Birthlight has an international network of specially trained yoga teachers who offer prenatal and postnatal yoga classes

British Wheel of Yoga
25, Jermyn Street, Sleaford, Lincolnshire NG34 7RU
Tel 01529 306851
www.bwy.org.uk
Email: office@bwy.org.uk
Umbrella organisation for the teaching of yoga in the UK

Yogabirth
www.yogabirth.org

MOTHER & BABY
National Childbirth Trust (NCT)
Alexandra House
Oldham Terrace, Acton
London W3 6NH
www.nctpregnancyandbabycare.com

La Leche League UK
BM3424, London, WC1N 3XX
Tel 020 7242 1278
www.laleche.org.uk

YOGA CLOTHES
Asquith Ltd
PO Box 31585, London, W11 1ZR
Tel 020 7792 8909
Fax: 020 7792 9414
www.asquith.ltd.uk
mail@asquith.ltd.uk

Jojo Maman Bebe Ltd
72 Bennerly Road
London, SW11 6DS
Tel 020 7924 3144

YOGA MATS & EQUIPMENT
Yoga Matters
32 Clarendon Road
London, N8 0DJ
Tel 020 8888 8588
www.yogamatters.com
Email: enquiries@yogamatters.com

CUSHIONED SUPPORTS etc
The White Company
Unit 30, Perivale Ind. Park
Horsenden Lane South
Greenford, Mddx, UB6 7RJ
Tel 0870 900 9555
www.thewhiteco.com

AUSTRALIA

Childbirth Education Association of Australia
www.cea-nsw.com.au
Email: info@cea-nsw.com.au

INDEX

ACKNOWLEDGMENTS

Author's acknowledgments

My first thanks go to my teachers of yoga and meditation. It has been a great joy to apply their insights, as my understanding gradually deepens, for the benefit of women in their journey towards motherhood. Many pregnant women, labouring women, new mothers and colleagues have inspired me. I cannot name them all, but special thanks go to Doriel Hall and Uma Dinsmore for their generous sharing of yoga; to Sally Lomas for her dedication to serving pregnant women and couples through Birthlight. I am also grateful to the Trustees of Birthlight, particularly to Margaret Adey, Elizabeth de Michelis, Diana Lomas, Frances Barnes and Regina Guilbride.

From photo-shoots with Russell Sadur to designing with Karen Sawyer and Sara Robin, this book has been produced by real DK teamwork, skilfully coordinated by Gillian Roberts, with a unique blend of professionalism, creative talent and sound humour. I would like to thank Claire Legemah for the beautiful design and Susannah Steel for her light approach to sensitive editing and her patience to the very end. Thanks to Mary-Clare Jerram for championing this book and to Robin Monro for giving perinatal yoga early recognition at the Yoga Biomedical Trust. Most of all, I wish to thank all the models for showing readers the positive benefits of yoga before and after birth. It has been a privilege to be part of Zac's birth.

Finally, this book is anchored in the loving support of my family at home, and, far away in Peru, in the legacy of the native grandmothers who taught me to give birth.

Publisher's acknowledgments

Dorling Kindersley would like to thank photographer Russell Sadur and his assistant, Nina Duncan; hair and make-up artist Toko; stylist Liz Hippsley; indexer Hilary Bird; models Helena Bryant, Katarina Gadjanski, Bergitte Heyer, Ann Hurst, Christina and Tony Susnjara, Natasha Rodan with Zion, Louise Powell with Lucas, Nasha and Jonathan Matin with Kaya, and Bergit Arends with Otto; and Jenny Lane for editorial assistance.

Special thanks to Asquith Ltd for supplying yoga clothes; Jojo Maman Bebe Ltd for supplying yoga and baby clothes; The White Company for loaning the suede cube, cushions and throws; and Yoga Matters for supplying the yoga mats and equipment.

ABOUT THE AUTHOR

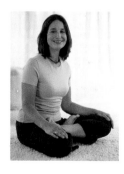

Françoise Barbira Freedman, PhD, is a medical anthropologist at Cambridge University. Her pioneering interest in pregnancy, childbirth and beyond stems from her earliest studies in the Amazon, where she was inspired by the energetic, light-hearted and gentle mothering of the Peruvian Amazonian women. An adept of yoga, she has used both her life experience as a mother of four and her academic training and research to develop her original approach to antenatal and postnatal holistic care.

Françoise has been a trainer for the Yoga Biomedical Trust's Yoga Therapist Diploma since 1994. She is a member of the Board of Yoga Therapists, which is developing professional standards for yoga therapy and guidelines for integration into NHS Trusts, and she also lectures at midwifery schools.

In 1990 Françoise founded the charity Birthlight, which is dedicated to promoting a sensitive approach to pregnancy, birth and babies through innovative applications of yoga and practical teachings across cultures. Birthlight offers classes in prenatal yoga, postnatal yoga, wellwoman yoga, yoga with babies and aquayoga for mothers and babies, as well as certificate and diploma courses in these subjects. The charity now has teachers and supporters in countries across Europe, North America, Latin America, Australia, New Zealand and the South Pacific.